Obesity Medicine:
Practice Tests

Obesity Medicine: Practice Tests

Kevin B. Smith, DO, FACP
ABOM Diplomate

300 Rapid Assessment Questions to Prepare for the American Board of Obesity Medicine Certification

2023 Edition

ISBN: 9798373588188

Independently published

Disclaimer: All efforts have been made to ensure accuracy and that the most up-to-date information is provided. Information in this review book should be used for study, not as a reference for patient care. It is up to the provider to ensure all information is accurate, and the author will not be held liable for inadvertent errors.

The item domains and rubrics for the Certification Examination for Obesity Medicine Physicians are available without charge on the ABOM website to facilitate individual study as well as review course development. The author of this review book has not been provided information regarding examination questions, nor does the author have preferential knowledge regarding actual questions included in the examination.

Copy editing performed by Kelly Smith

For correspondence, including questions, concerns, or errata, please contact: obesitymedicinereview@gmail.com

Free weekly study blogs, book updates, and discounts can be found at obesitymedicinereview.com or by scanning QR code.

Practice Test 1

1. A patient with end-stage renal disease on hemodialysis is presenting to a bariatric clinic for weight loss to become eligible for a renal transplant. Medications are discussed in detail. Which is the most appropriate treatment to start at this time?

    A. Semaglutide
    B. Naltrexone/buproprion ER
    C. Phentermine/topiramate ER
    D. Cellulose and Citric Acid Hydrogel

2. A patient presents to a dermatologist with follicular hyperkeratosis. She had a malabsorptive procedure six years ago and admits to poor nutritional intake. Which vitamin or mineral, if replaced, would most likely improve her symptoms?

    A. Vitamin A
    B. Vitamin E
    C. Zinc
    D. Selenium

3. A patient takes supplemental folate. Where is the location of absorption for this vitamin?

    A. Duodenum
    B. Jejunum
    C. Ileum
    D. Colon

4. A 44-year-old female undergoes a workup for delayed post-prandial hypoglycemia two years after undergoing a gastric bypass. She is ultimately diagnosed with hyperinsulinemic hypoglycemia due to islet cell hypertrophy and undergoes dietary changes without an improvement in symptoms. Which class of medications is indicated?

    A. Complex disaccharides
    B. Beta-blockers
    C. Sulfonylureas
    D. Biguanides

5. A 49-year-old male underwent a Roux-en-Y gastric bypass two years prior. He has taken vitamins intermittently. His vitamin D level is low and appropriate supplementation is initiated. What should be his maintenance dose?

A. 1000 IU daily
B. 2000 IU daily
C. 50000 IU weekly
D. A dose to maintain levels > 30 ng/mL

6. A 44-year-old female consumes 40% of her calories in the evening when she returns home from work. In the morning, she denies hunger and often skips breakfast. What other finding is most likely present?

A. Sense of lack of control over eating
B. Increased dietary carbohydrate: protein ratio
C. Parasomnia
D. Purging behaviors after eating episodes

7. A 29-year-old female has completed her bariatric evaluation and is planning to undergo a sleeve gastrectomy within the next six months. She is currently on oral contraceptives. When should her contraceptive pills be stopped before surgery?

A. Right now
B. One month prior
C. One week prior
D. Continue these perioperatively

8. A 21-year-old female presents to the clinic for evaluation of an IUD placement. Poor dentition and calluses over her knuckles are noted on the physical exam. She appears withdrawn and does not want to discuss other preventative measures. Which of the following statements is most accurate regarding her underlying condition?

A. Prevalence is equal among males and females
B. There are no FDA-approved pharmacologic treatments
C. BMIs are often in the underweight range
D. Patients have a higher prevalence of prior sexual abuse

9. A 7-year-old boy with a history of leptin deficiency is treated with appropriate medication. Two months later, he returns to the clinic, and his weight is reduced by 20 lbs (9.1 kg). Which of the following central hormones was likely inhibited after the initiation of treatment?

A. Proopiomelanocortin
B. Alpha melanocyte-stimulating hormone
C. Cocaine and amphetamine-regulated transcript
D. Orexin A and B

10. A physician works alongside a physician assistant (PA) in a busy primary care clinic. The PA notices that most of the patients the physician assigns to him for the day have a BMI > 40 kg/m², whereas the patients the physician sees are generally of a normal BMI. The physician seems unaware of this pattern. This is an example of which of the following principles?

A. Prejudice
B. Stigma
C. Implicit bias
D. Malpractice

11. A 39-year-old patient presents to a family practice clinic with complaints of brittle hair and cold intolerance. She has a history of hypothyroidism but has been stable on her dose for three years. She does admit to going to a weight loss clinic and being prescribed an anti-obesity medication. Which of the following weight-loss medications explains her presenting symptoms?

A. Orlistat
B. Semaglutide
C. Phentermine
D. Buproprion ER

12. For a small cost, a kiosk at the mall measures body fat percentages via bioelectrical impedance analysis (BIA) or calipers. Which of the following patients should BIA be recommended for testing over calipers?

A. BMI > 45 kg/m^2
B. Presence of a cardiac pacemaker
C. Patient with decompensated cirrhosis
D. Patient with poor skin turgor

13. A 43-year-old female with class III obesity is referred to the lymphedema clinic. Her lower extremity physical examination findings most likely include which of the following?

A. Cuff sign
B. "Round pea" sensation
C. Stemmer's sign
D. Lipodystrophy

14. A 54-year-old male has made many dietary changes in the past year. He denies having time for physical activity but states his job "keeps him active." He has lost nearly 35 lbs (15.9 kg) during this time. He says he recently felt more hungry and has started to graze in the evenings. This has caused nearly 10 lbs (4.5 kg) in weight regain during the past two months. What mechanism is likely the culprit for his recent weight changes?

A. Neurohurmonal influences
B. Adaptive thermogenesis
C. Set-point fallacy
D. Increased muscle efficiency

15. A patient asks about realistic expectations that could be obtained after a Roux-en-Y gastric bypass. The average percentage of total body weight loss in 1 year is approximately

A. 20-25%
B. 25-30%
C. 30-35%
D. 35-40%

16. Which is the most appropriate way to obtain the most accurate blood pressure?

    A. Rest the arm comfortably by the side
    B. Ensure clothes underneath the cuff is not bunched up
    C. The cuff bladder should encircle 80% of the arm circumference
    D. Distract the patient by talking with them

17. A 4-year-old with excess weight is being evaluated. When reviewing the chart, it is noted that the patient was treated in the NICU after birth due to profound hypotension. This patient most likely carries a defect in which gene?

    A. Proopiomelanocortin
    B. Leptin receptor
    C. Melanocortin receptor
    D. Orexin gene

18. Which of the following comorbidities should be treated with bupropion in a patient with excess weight?

    A. General anxiety disorder
    B. Alcohol use disorder
    C. Tics
    D. Seasonal affective disorder

19. A 19-year-old female has recently been diagnosed with body dysmorphic syndrome. She states it is related to the excess adipose tissue on her stomach, of which she was bullied in high school by students telling her she looked pregnant. Since then, she has joined a gym and works on abdominal crunches for 2 hours daily. Which of the following is consistent with her condition?

    A. Constantly asking friends for their opinions on her abdomen
    B. Avoidance of mirrors or viewing herself in pictures
    C. Preoccupation with other peoples' similarly enlarged abdomens
    D. Diagnosis of concurrent bulimia nervosa

20. Which of the following is the most accurate mechanism of ghrelin?

A. Stimulates NPY/AgRP receptors
B. Suppresses gut motility to promote absorption
C. Increases energy expenditure
D. Stimulates insulin secretion

21. Which of the following findings is more characteristic of an anastomotic ulcer when compared to a stricture following a Roux-en-Y gastric bypass?

A. Diagnosis involves an upper barium evaluation
B. Treatment includes endoscopic procedures
C. Pain is more localized within the abdomen
D. Symptoms can progress to dysphagia

22. A patient who admits to being addicted to soda is recently started on a medication to help with soda aversion, as it alters carbonic anhydrase on the tongue. What is the mechanism of this medication?

A. Stimulation of the hypothalamus to release norepinephrine
B. Enhancement of GABA activity and sodium channels
C. Agonist of glucagon-like 1 peptide receptor
D. Neuronal reuptake inhibition of norepinephrine and dopamine

23. A 34-year-old businessman presents for therapy following a psychiatric evaluation. He is pursuing the gastric sleeve to cut down on the large meals he eats in a short duration of time. He admits he becomes embarrassed when he finishes his meal before his colleagues at meetings. What condition does he likely meet the criteria for?

A. Night eating syndrome
B. Major depressive disorder
C. Binge eating disorder
D. Body dysmorphic syndrome

24. OARS is an acronym used in the setting of motivational interviewing. What does the 'R' stand for in this acronym?

A. Reiterate
B. Rapport
C. Reflection
D. Readiness

25. A patient classified as stage 3 on the Edmonton Obesity Staging System (EOSS) would likely have which of the following comorbidities?

A. Suicidal ideation related to weight
B. Hypertension
C. End-stage renal disease from diabetes
D. Pre-diabetes

26. Which of the following is considered an autosomal recessive cause of early-onset childhood obesity?

A. Congenital leptin deficiency
B. Prader-Willi syndrome
C. MC4R deficiency
D. Beckwith-Wiedemann syndrome

27. The rate of those diagnosed with excess weight continues to increase in the American population. Which of the following statements is most accurate?

A. 70% of adults have a BMI ≥ 30 kg/m^2
B. 1 in 3 children have obesity
C. 4 out of 10 adults meet the criteria for obesity
D. Rates of class III obesity has decreased in children

28. A 22-year-old presents to the emergency department by the police due to concerns about an inability to care for herself. She weighs 79 lbs (35.8 kg) and is concerned that she weighs too much. She has only consumed one large vegan salad daily for the past six months. What is likely seen on examination?

A. Abdominal fluid wave
B. Folate deficiency
C. Vitamin C deficiency
D. Tachycardia

29. A 64-year-old female underwent a laparoscopic adjustable gastric banding (LABG) 6 years prior and has had minimal follow-up. She now states that she is having considerable abdominal pain. She says she can eat whatever she wants without feeling full. On physical examination, the port site appears red, with purulence noted. Which of the following is the most likely diagnosis?

A. Anastomotic leak
B. Band erosion
C. Gastric pouch dilation
D. Band slippage

30. A 33-year-old female presents with facial plethora and new-onset diabetes. On physical examination, she has a dorsal fat pad. Which of the following is the most critical next step in determining the etiology of her presentation?

A. Medication review
B. Cancer screening
C. Adrenal imaging
D. Dexamethasone suppression testing

31. A patient successfully underwent a Roux-en-Y gastric bypass but now has recurrent episodes of tachycardia, facial flushing, abdominal cramping, and diarrhea after eating larger meals. What is the best next step for this patient?

    A. Screen for undiagnosed carcinoid syndrome
    B. Avoidance of foods with high concentrations of fats
    C. Increase protein intake
    D. Perform a breath hydrogen test

32. A patient was recently diagnosed with binge eating disorder. The only FDA medication specifically approved for this condition is also approved for which of the following?

    A. Depression
    B. Chronic migraines
    C. Untreated obstructive sleep apnea
    D. Attention deficit disorder

33. What is the respiratory quotient of proteins?

    A. 0.7
    B. 0.8
    C. 1
    D. 1.2

34. A patient with previously poor nutrition decides to increase fiber intake with both dietary supplements and an increased intake of vegetables and fruits. What effect is this likely to have?

    A. Resolution or improvement of acne
    B. Improvements in cholesterol
    C. Increased desire for energy-dense foods
    D. Decreased risk of atrial fibrillation

35. An example of primary prevention for the development of obesity would include which of the following options?

    A. Providing behavioral therapy interventions in an obesity clinic
    B. Supplying free dietary plans for those with sleep apnea
    C. Presenting pharmacotherapy options at a bariatric seminar
    D. Sponsoring a day camp for youth focused on physical activity

36. A 13-year-old male with class II obesity presents with a limp with walking. He states he has been trying to exercise more but is limited by his pain. He is diagnosed with slipped capital femoral epiphysis. What would likely be seen on x-ray imaging?

    A. Salter-Harris fracture
    B. Bowing of the tibia
    C. Avascular necrosis of the femoral head
    D. Increased ossification of the tibial tuberosity

37. A 73-year-old female wants to start an exercise and dietary plan after a "wake-up call" with a recent myocardial infarction. Which of the following would be most appropriate to recommend as part of her regimen to prevent sarcopenia?

    A. One hundred grams of protein intake daily
    B. Total calorie intake of ≤ 1200 kcal/day
    C. Daily aerobic stationary bicycle riding
    D. Calcium and vitamin D supplementation

38. Theoretically, a person who has a normal body mass index, when compared to a person with an elevated BMI, has increased levels of which of the following in the gastrointestinal tract?

    A. Prebiotic secretion
    B. Energy harvesting
    C. Bacteroides
    D. Firmicutes

39. A 19-year-old female is brought into the emergency department after passing out during a competitive dance competition. On arrival, she is alert and oriented, has poor skin turgor, and has temporal wasting. Her heart rate is 52/min. Based on the most likely diagnosis, which other findings would be appreciated?

    A. Lack of concern about her low weight
    B. Body mass index of 19 kg/m^2
    C. Peaked T waves on an electrocardiogram
    D. Pitting edema and anasarca

40. A pediatrician diagnoses a male patient with a condition similar to binge eating disorder seen in adult patients. Which of the following characteristics is likely present in this patient?

    A. Apathy regarding his eating patterns
    B. Tanner Stage 2
    C. Purging after large meals
    D. Symptoms ongoing for two months

41. A laboratory monitors caloric utilization by different organ systems. Of the following, which would have the highest caloric requirements in a resting individual?

    A. Heart
    B. Kidney
    C. Fat
    D. Brain

42. A 28-year-old female presents to discuss her prior weight loss attempts. She states she drinks four sodas daily and eats out almost daily for convenience. She says she finds it impossible to imagine not having these eating patterns. Which of the following phrases would be most appropriate at his time?

    A. Why do you think you cannot change?
    B. It sounds like you need some family support
    C. You seem motivated to make some changes
    D. Why do you drink that much soda in a day?

43. A 24-year-old previously healthy female begins exercising 2-3 hours per day to gain muscle mass. She eats 6-12 raw egg whites daily for increased protein. If she continues this regimen, which vitamin deficiency is she most prone to develop?

A. Thiamine
B. Riboflavin
C. Biotin
D. Folate

44. During an esophagogastroduodenoscopy, a biopsy of the duodenum is completed. Specialized testing reveals an anorexic hormone secreted from the K-cells. What hormone is being secreted?

A. Glucagon-like peptide 1
B. Cholecystokinin
C. Peptide YY
D. Glucose-dependent insulinotropic peptide

45. A patient underwent a successful laparoscopic Roux-en-Y gastric bypass and is 8 hours post-operative. The nurse notices darker urine despite adequate intraoperative fluid administration. Which intraoperative risk factors likely contributed to this patient's condition?

A. Length of surgery
B. Biliary duct injury
C. Traumatic Foley insertion
D. Reaction to medications

46. A pediatrician is interested in prescribing medications for weight loss. Based on her comfort level, she does not want to prescribe any medications off-label. Which of the following weight-loss medications would be an option for her?

A. Metformin in a 12-year-old
B. Liraglutide in a teenager
C. Phentermine for a 6-month duration in a 17-year-old
D. Naltrexone/bupropion ER in a 15-year-old

47. A psychiatrist is treating a patient with new-onset bipolar disorder. The patient has class II obesity and is concerned about medication-induced weight gain. Which of the following is the most weight-neutral mood stabilizer?

A. Divalproex
B. Lithium
C. Gabapentin
D. Lamotrigine

48. A 9-year-old male presents to a multidisciplinary weight loss center. Laboratory work will be obtained during this visit. When would it be most appropriate to obtain liver enzymes to screen for metabolic-associated fatty liver disease (MAFLD)?

A. If the patient's weight is in the 90th percentile with a diagnosis of prediabetes
B. On any patient with a BMI greater than the 85th percentile
C. Regardless of BMI, if the parents have a history of metabolic-associated
D. If the patient's weight is at the 94th percentile

49. How would ursodeoxycholic acid be used in the management of patients with obesity?

A. To prevent the progression of fatty liver disease
B. Dissolve formed gallstones after bariatric surgery
C. To treat dumping syndrome post Roux-en-Y gastric bypass
D. Prevent cholecystectomy after gastric bypass surgery

50. Using growth charts based on the percentile of body mass index is best in which of the following cohorts?

A. Neonatal period
B. Once a child begins walking
C. Those over the age of 2
D. Tanner Stage 2 and above

Practice Test 2

51. A 51-year-old female presents for her annual evaluation after undergoing a successful Roux-en-Y gastric bypass three years prior. She states that she has had frequent yeast infections within the skin folds of her abdomen despite trying to keep them clean and dry. Which of the following is the most appropriate solution to this problem?

A. Oral fluconazole
B. Topical nystatin cream
C. Referral to plastic surgery
D. Topical clindamycin

52. A patient was recently started on topiramate for idiopathic intracranial hypertension and weight loss (off-label). Which of the following lab abnormalities is expected with topiramate use?

A. Elevated triglycerides
B. Non-anion gap metabolic acidosis
C. Lactic acidosis
D. Hyperkalemia

53. The most common long-term complication of laparoscopic adjustable gastric banding is

A. band slippage
B. erosion
C. port issues
D. required revision/removal

54. A 36-year-old male presents to the emergency department with jaundice and darkened urine. On laboratory analysis, he is found to be in acute hepatic failure. He states he started a supplement that was supposed to help with increasing energy expenditure. Which of the following is most likely contributing to his presentation?

A. Yerba Mate
B. Guar gum
C. Chitosan
D. Hydroxycitric acid

55. A patient starts cellulose and citric acid hydrogel to assist with weight loss. The hydrated capsules will eventually break down in the gastrointestinal tract, with water reabsorption occurring at what location?

 A. Duodenum
 B. Jejunum
 C. Ileum
 D. Colon

56. A 44-year-old male underwent a sleeve gastrectomy complicated by prior surgical adhesions and scarring, requiring conversion to an open surgery. Given the additional time for stomach resection, the surgery time lengthened significantly. Which of the following is likely to be increased on post-operative day one?

 A. Bicarbonate level
 B. Creatine phosphokinase
 C. Sodium and chloride
 D. Total bilirubin

57. A pediatric clinic is starting a weight management program where they can provide support through dieticians and physical therapists to provide motivational interviewing and monthly follow-up visits. Which of the following accurately describes the highest-tiered intervention they can provide?

 A. Prevention
 B. Prevention plus
 C. Structured weight management
 D. Comprehensive multidisciplinary intervention

58. A patient is establishing care with a new primary care physician. It is noted that metformin is on his medication list without a diagnosis of diabetes. The patient states that his psychiatrist started a medication that may cause weight gain and simultaneously prescribed metformin to reduce that side effect. What other medicine was this patient likely prescribed?

A. Olanzapine
B. Nortriptyline
C. Bupropion
D. Desvenlafaxine

59. After discussing weight loss goals and preferences, a patient is encouraged to develop a SMART goal. In this acronym, what does the 'M' stand for?

A. Measurable
B. Meaningful
C. Motivation
D. Manageable

60. A 47-year-old female with hyperlipidemia and prediabetes presents to her primary care physician because she is not tolerating statin therapy. She would prefer to pursue dietary modifications rather than medication for primary cardiovascular prevention. She is planning to start on a low-carbohydrate or keto diet. Three months from now, how will her laboratory work change?

A. Decreased HDL
B. Increase in TG
C. Increase in LDL
D. Unchanged total cholesterol

61. A patient is being treated with cognitive behavioral therapy for a condition in which she eats excessively in a short amount of time and then has immense guilt. She hides her behaviors from her friends. Which of the following therapies would most likely be beneficial to her?

A. Topiramate
B. Buspirone
C. Bariatric surgery
D. Semaglutide

62. A 21-year-old female presents to her primary care for follow-up regarding prior insulin resistance. She was recently started on metformin and initiated lifestyle changes. She has lost 2% of her body weight but states her menstrual cycles are still irregular. Which of the following findings was most likely present on her initial evaluation?

A. Dorsal fat pad
B. Unilateral adnexal enlargement
C. Seborrheic keratosis
D. Adrenergic alopecia

63. A patient who underwent a successful Roux-en-Y gastric bypass presents for a one-month post-operative follow-up appointment. Although the patient has experienced weight loss, she states she is now unable to tolerate solid food and has reverted to a liquid diet. She felt like food was getting stuck. Which of the following is the most appropriate treatment for her condition?

A. Antibiotics
B. Endoscopic procedure
C. Anti-inflammatories
D. Laparoscopic revision

64. Patients with which of the following conditions should consistently utilize special growth charts and BMI curves?

A. Down syndrome
B. Addison's disease
C. Achondroplasia
D. Congenital hypothyroidism

65. Which of the following is an essential amino acid?

A. Arginine
B. Methionine
C. Proline
D. Tyrosine

66. A nurse tells a physician that she received a call regarding one of his patients that was not tolerating one of her new blood pressure medications. The patient's BMI is 46 kg/m². The physician states, "She probably just doesn't want to take medicines; she never does anything I tell her." This attitude is an example of which of the following?

A. Stigma
B. Burnout
C. Implicit bias
D. Prejudice

67. A 39-year-old male presents six months after a sleeve gastrectomy with complaints of debilitating gastroesophageal reflux in the evenings. He has tried dietary changes, sleeping in a recliner, and increasing omeprazole to twice daily without relief. A urease breath test and barium study is unremarkable. Which of the following would be appropriate at this time?

A. Add famotidine to his medicine regimen
B. Evaluate for a hiatal hernia with endoscopy
C. Initiate metoclopramide before meals
D. Conversion to a Roux-en-Y gastric bypass

68. A 44-year-old female with class III obesity presents to her primary care physician to review recent test results for daytime fatigue. She has hypertension controlled with chlorthalidone. She underwent a home polysomnography which showed no desaturations and minimal apneic events. Her blood work revealed significant respiratory acidosis. Her echocardiogram revealed minimally elevated right ventricular pressures without other abnormalities. Which of the following is the best next step in management?

A. Trial a non-invasive positive airway pressure machine
B. Repeat the polysomnography at a sleep facility
C. Order pulmonary function testing
D. Evaluate with a right heart catheterization

69. A 19-year-old female presents to her primary care physician with the chief complaint of "being funny-shaped." In particular, she complains of needing to shop for larger pant sizes, but her shoe size is relatively small. What additional finding would be most likely?

A. Abdominal striae and easy bruising
B. History of lymph node dissection
C. Similar exam findings in her sister
D. Telangiectasias and caput medussa

70. A patient presents with decreased sensation to monofilament testing and reduced vibratory sensations in the lower extremity bilaterally. These findings may be seen in which of the following water-soluble vitamin deficiencies?

A. B_2
B. B_3
C. B_6
D. B_9

71. A company produces a synthetic high-potency hormone that suppresses glucagon production and increases satiety. What of the following hormones does this describe?

    A. Cholecystokinin
    B. Peptide YY
    C. Oxyntomodulin
    D. Glucagon-like peptide 1

72. A 12-year-old female presents for a well-child visit. Which is the most accurate way of classifying her weight category?

    A. Weight-for-length
    B. Absolute BMI
    C. Percentile range of BMI
    D. Percentage of body fat

73. A 19-year-old male with obesity presents for dietary counseling. He admits to working longer hours during the day and frequently snacks on potato chips, peanut butter sandwiches, and soda. When he gets home, he eats a significant amount of calories throughout the evening and occasionally wakes up in the night for a quick snack. Which of the following recommendations would have the most significant impact on his eating habits?

    A. Eat breakfast every morning
    B. Increase unsaturated fat intake to slow gastric emptying
    C. Begin pharmacotherapy with phentermine
    D. Change to wholegrain bread

74. In the setting of low-energy sustainable exercise (such as a slow jog in a marathon), if a steady state is maintained, the respiratory quotient will predominantly indicate burning which of the following elements?

    A. Carbohydrates
    B. Proteins
    C. Fats
    D. Fruits

75. A couple decides to pursue a diet that avoids poultry and red meat. However, they plan to continue to eat salmon and almond milk. Which of the following diets does this describe?

    A. Lacto-ova
    B. Pescatarian
    C. Vegan
    D. Vegetarian

76. What is the benefit of utilizing the Edmonton Obesity Staging System (EOSS) over anthropometric measurements such as waist circumference and body mass index (BMI)?

    A. It is used to screen candidates for obstructive sleep apnea
    B. Life insurance companies use it to determine surgery eligibility
    C. It helps determine the long-term impact of obesity on a patient
    D. It justifies bariatric surgery in those who do not meet BMI criteria

77. A 16-year-old male is brought into the clinic for concerns of an eating disorder. Which of the following would best differentiate the eating disorder of bulimia from anorexia?

    A. Fear of gaining weight
    B. Compensatory behaviors
    C. Body mass index
    D. Self-image distortion

78. A 51-year-old male presents with peripheral vision loss, headaches, and decreased sexual desire. Subsequent imaging shows a cystic structure in the pituitary stalk. Which of the following best describes this finding?

    A. Prolactinoma
    B. Pituitary macroadenoma
    C. Craniopharyngioma
    D. Optic glioma

79. A 29-year-old female is presenting for a one-week follow-up after undergoing a successful Roux-en-Y gastric bypass. Although she has discontinued her sliding scale insulin due to a hypoglycemic episode, she has had persistent post-prandial hyperglycemia of 180-200 mg/dL. Her medications for diabetes currently include metformin ER and maximally tolerated semaglutide. Which of the following would be the best pharmacologic management of her diabetes?

A. Resume a reduced insulin sliding scale
B. Stop metformin due to the risk of lactic acidosis
C. Change the metformin formulation
D. Initiate and up-titrate empagliflozin

80. Which antipsychotic medication would be most appropriate for a patient with excess weight?

A. Olanzapine
B. Ariprazole
C. Clozapine
D. Risperidone

81. A pharmacy receives a shipment of metreleptin. Which patient diagnosis is an indication for this therapy?

A. Proopiomelanocortin gene mutations
B. Congenital leptin deficiency
C. PCSK1 genetic defect
D. Melanocortin 4 receptor deficiency

82. A patient begins a new exercise program utilizing boxing for cardiac aerobic therapy. The type of muscle fibers used in this program have which of the following properties?

A. Has significantly higher levels of mitochondria
B. Tends to be fatigue-resistant
C. Is similar to the muscles used in triathlons
D. Uses anaerobic glycolysis for metabolism

24

83. An aspiration device is being offered at a bariatric surgery clinic. A patient with the following conditions would be a poor candidate to receive this therapy?

A. Body mass index of 51 kg/m^2
B. Significant mental disability
C. A history of multiple C-sections
D. Paraplegia of lower extremities

84. An endogenous rectal hormone is synthetically produced and injected into mice. The mice have transient gastroparesis and increase the length of time between feedings. What hormone is being described?

A. Glucagon-like peptide 1
B. Oxyntomodulin
C. Peptide YY
D. Leptin

85. A 52-year-old male has been waking up in the middle of the night to eat food while still asleep. This has occurred approximately three times weekly over the past three months. The patient is most likely to have which of the following findings?

A. Periodic limb movement disorder
B. Orthostatic hypotension
C. Use of fluoxetine
D. Family history of dementia

86. A zinc deficiency could cause which of the following symptoms?

A. Anemia
B. Night blindness
C. Seborrheic dermatitis
D. Anosmia

87. A 2-year-old male with gross motor deficits presents with his parents to a nutritionist after recently gaining weight. Genetic testing reveals a paternal chromosome 15q partial deletion. Which of the following would likely be seen upon examining his hands?

   A. Normal fingers
   B. Polydactyly
   C. Shortened 4th and 5th metacarpal bones
   D. Brachydactyly

88. An obesity medicine specialist meets with a new patient interested in behavioral modification related to weight loss. The physician states, "I understand it can be difficult to lose weight. Tell me about your history with trying to lose weight?" Which key process of motivational interviewing is being displayed?

   A. Evoking
   B. Planning
   C. Engagement
   D. Focusing

89. The two most commonly acquired information for obesity rates and statistics is based on surveys from the National Health and Nutrition Examination Survey (NHANES) and the Behavioral Risk Factor Surveillance System (BRFSS). Which of the following statements on obesity surveying is most accurate?

   A. BRFSS surveys are based on a larger sample size
   B. NHANES surveys are based on self-reported weight data
   C. BRFSS has consistently been more accurate with weight
   D. NHANES surveys tend to over-report rates of obesity

90. A 44-year-old female presents to the clinic after losing nearly 13 lbs (5.9 kg) within the last three months. Her weight has been stable over the past five years before this recent weight loss. When would her level of sex hormone binding globulin (SHBG) be highest?

A. Now
B. Three months ago
C. Three years ago
D. Five years ago

91. What is most accurate regarding the cohort data from the Centers for Disease Control and Prevention (CDC) growth charts?

A. Data is based predominantly on breastfed children
B. These charts best reflect those between 0-2 years of age
C. The CDC charts should not be utilized in other countries
D. Data is based predominantly on Caucasians

92. A 34-year-old female is interested in starting phentermine/topiramate ER after not meeting weight loss goals with lifestyle modifications alone. What would be the best question to ask before initiating this medication?

A. Can you remember to take medications twice daily?
B. Have you had any previous seizures?
C. Are you on any chronic pain medications?
D. Are you sexually active?

93. A patient is brought to the operating room before undergoing a sleeve gastrectomy procedure. The anesthesiologist finds out that the patient had a meal replacement shake 3 hours before the surgery and threatens to cancel the surgery. Which of the following would be the best response?

A. "I agree. This patient is at high risk for aspiration."
B. "The shake will help with post-operative bowel function."
C. "If the shake was clear, it should be okay to continue with surgery."
D. "Let's delay surgery for a few more hours."

94. A 24-year-old female presents to the clinic for follow-up after starting an FDA-approved anti-obesity medication that causes decreased fat absorption. What is a potential complication of this medication?

    A. Thiamine deficiency
    B. Congenital birth defects
    C. Nephrolithiasis
    D. Cholelithiasis

95. An 11-year-old female presents to her pediatrician for a follow-up regarding weight management. The patient's weight is in the 95th percentile, and blood pressure was elevated on the prior visit. Her mother has end-stage cirrhosis secondary to metabolic-associated liver disease (MAFLD). Given the above findings, what is the best initial screening test for this patient?

    A. AST: ALT ratio
    B. ALT
    C. AST
    D. MAFLD fibrosis score

96. A 14-year-old adolescent with an arm circumference of 32 cm presents for a blood pressure evaluation. His blood pressure was elevated during a prior examination, although ambulatory home measurements were within normal limits. Which of the following cuff sizes is most appropriate for this patient?

    A. Pediatric (18-22 cm)
    B. Small adult (22-26 cm)
    C. Adult (27-34 cm)
    D. Large adult (45-52 cm)

97. Which of the following is most similar to loss of control eating disorder?

    A. Bulimia Nervosa
    B. Night eating syndrome
    C. Leptin deficiency
    D. Binge eating disorder

98. Education is being provided to new foster parents of a 5-year-old regarding maintaining a healthy weight. Which of the following recommendations is most appropriate?

    A. Limit sugar-sweetened beverages to no more than one per day
    B. Breakfast should be limited to oatmeal, fruits, or eggs
    C. An hour of physical activity is recommended daily
    D. Children with 7-8 hours of sleep perform optimally during school

99. The orexigenic hormone produced in the stomach would be at its peak levels in which scenario?

    A. With increased adipose tissue
    B. After the consumption of carbohydrates
    C. Status post sleeve gastrectomy
    D. During a stressed state

100. A 33-year-old Caucasian male presents to his primary care physician after gaining 45 lbs (20.4 kg) over the past year since working from home. His blood pressure has been persistently elevated, and he is agreeable to starting an anti-hypertensive medication while working on lifestyle changes. Which class of antihypertensive should be recommended?

    A. Calcium channel blocker
    B. Thiazide diuretic
    C. Beta-blocker
    D. Angiotensin receptor blocker

Practice Test 3

101. An 18-year-old female presents to her primary care physician for persistent headaches and occasional double vision. She states these occurred toward the end of her first semester of college. Since graduating high school, she has gained approximately 25 lbs (11.3 kg). Her eye doctor noted abnormalities on fundoscopic examination, although her corrective lenses are adequate. Her STOP-BANG score is 2. Which of the following is the most appropriate treatment?

A. Counseling regarding alcohol use
B. Carbonic anhydrase inhibitors
C. CPAP machine at night
D. Latanoprost eye drops

102. Cellulose and citric acid hydrogel (brand name Plenity®) is approved for what minimum body mass index with no obesity-related comorbidity?

A. 23 kg/m^2
B. 25 kg/m^2
C. 27 kg/m^2
D. 30 kg/m^2

103. A 59-year-old male presents to the emergency department due to dehydration and lack of oral nutrition. He is eight months status-post Roux-en-Y gastric bypass. He has lost nearly 85 lbs (38.6 kg) post-operatively but has developed intermittent abdominal pain and post-prandial satiety over the past two months. Over the last two days, his abdominal pain significantly increased, and he could not tolerate any oral intake. A CT scan shows a mesenteric swirl sign. Which of the following is the most likely diagnosis?

A. Large bowel obstruction
B. Volvulus
C. Small bowel ileus
D. Internal hernia

104. A 37-year-old patient is considering quitting smoking within the next month. He wanted to discuss strategies that are used to help with the process. This patient is most likely in which of the following stages of change?

A. Pre-contemplation
B. Contemplation
C. Preparation
D. Action

105. A patient has been recommended to undergo tarsal tunnel surgery, but the podiatrist will not perform the surgery until the patient has lost 5% of his weight. The patient has not lost enough weight with extensive lifestyle changes alone and wishes to discuss weight loss options, including placing a gastric balloon. Which of the following recommendations is most appropriate?

A. Plan for tarsal tunnel surgery six months after the balloon is placed
B. The balloon is unlikely to reduce weight by 5%
C. A BMI of 34 kg/m^2 does not meet the criteria for a balloon
D. If used appropriately, balloons have a high risk of deflation and bowel obstruction

106. A 34-year-old female underwent a bariatric surgery complicated by intrabdominal adhesions from prior C-sections and laparoscopic cholecystectomy. The patient is difficult to wean from the ventilator, with oxygen desaturations and increased respiratory rate when placed on spontaneous breathing. Which of the following is the most likely cause?

A. Venous thromboembolism
B. Obesity hypoventilation syndrome
C. Obstructive sleep apnea
D. Rhabdomyolysis

107. During a weight management discussion, a physician documents a weight loss plan, including specific goals discussed during the visit. Which action does this describe based on the 5 A's of obesity management?

A. Assess
B. Advise
C. Agree
D. Assist

108. Indirect calorimetry would best help determine which of the following metabolic parameters?

A. Resting energy expenditure
B. Non-exercise activity thermogenesis
C. Thermic effect of meals
D. Energy expenditure from physical activity

109. A female presents to her primary care physician with numbness and weakness in the lower extremities. Physical examination reveals an abnormal gait with sensory ataxia. What nutritional deficiency does this describe?

A. Riboflavin
B. Copper
C. Niacin
D. Zinc

110. A psychologist is using motivational interviewing skills in a multidisciplinary obesity medicine clinic. The patient has lost 10 lbs (4.5 kg) in the past four weeks but does admit to still eating fast food 1-2 times weekly. Which of the following statements or questions reflect the principle of supporting self-efficacy?

A. "What can you do to maintain this rate of weight loss in the future?"
B. "Your weight loss could be even more impressive if you avoided fast food."
C. "Your weight loss in the past four weeks shows your motivation."
D. "What skills do you think were most influential in your successful weight loss?"

111. A biologist is studying relative hormone levels secreted by adipose tissue. It is determined that the most abundant hormone synthesized and released by adipose tissue

    A. increases aromatase conversion of estrogen
    B. enhances insulin sensitivity and skeletal glucose uptake
    C. increases inflammation within the vascular endothelium
    D. slows down gastrointestinal motility

112. Which of the following is a contraindication for metformin use?

    A. Prior Roux-en-Y gastric bypass
    B. Concurrent diastolic heart failure
    C. A patient over the age of 70 years old
    D. A patient on peritoneal dialysis

113. Which of the following hormones is a long-acting signaling hormone that increases in the setting of excess adiposity?

    A. Orexin
    B. Leptin
    C. Adiponectin
    D. Glucagon

114. Naltrexone/bupropion ER should be avoided in patients with which of the following characteristics?

    A. A history of opioid use disorder
    B. A blood pressure of 160/90 mmHg
    C. A history of calcium oxalate nephrolithiasis
    D. A history of depression

115. An 11-year-old female with a diagnosis of obesity class I presents to her pediatrician at her mother's urging. For the past six months, she has been stashing a significant amount of food in her room and rapidly eating it. The rest of the day, she looks defeated and is very irritable. Which of the following is the most effective management for her likely condition?

A. Psychotherapy
B. Metformin
C. Topiramate
D. Group therapy

116. A radiotracer with an affinity to orexin is injected during a molecular study. Where is the location the tracer is most likely to accumulate?

A. Arcuate nucleus
B. Lateral hypothalamic area
C. Paraventricular nucleus
D. Melanocortin 3 and 4 receptors

117. A mother brings her 17-year-old daughter in for evaluation after recently finding that she has trouble focusing throughout the day. She stays up late and has difficulty falling asleep. The patient was recently started on medication to help with weight loss which she takes daily with lunch. The medication the patient was most likely started on has a mechanism most similar to which of the following?

A. Zonisomide
B. Dulaglutide
C. Diethylpropion
D. Verenacylcine

118. A patient is interested in a low-fat diet due to hypercholesterolemia and a prior myocardial infarction. This diet is sustained for six months. Although the patient denies significant weight loss, he feels better and admits to having more energy. If labs are obtained today, which of the following would likely improve the most?

    A. LDL cholesterol
    B. HbA1c levels
    C. Triglycerides
    D. Total cholesterol

119. A 55-year-old female presents to the clinic regarding significant insomnia interfering with her quality of life. She has tried melatonin, sleep hygiene, and cognitive behavioral therapy without success. Zaleplon is prescribed short-term. Which condition is associated with this medication?

    A. Binge eating disorder
    B. Anti-psychotic induced weight gain
    C. Sleep-related eating disorder
    D. Night eating syndrome

120. A recent medication has been found to increase adipose tissue that contains significantly more mitochondria. If studied further, this adipose tissue would display what quality?

    A. Mechanically inefficient
    B. Reduces core body temperature
    C. Promotes energy expenditure through shivering
    D. Suppresses metabolic rate proportionately

121. A patient who has undergone a sleeve gastrectomy is most likely to have which of the following direct neurohormonal responses?

    A. Activation of the POMC/CART pathway
    B. Inhibition of the NPY/AgRP
    C. Decreased activation of the NPY/AgRP
    D. Suppression of the POMC/CART pathway

122. Glucagon-like peptide 1 is secreted by what cell type in the small intestines?

A. I-cells
B. K-cells
C. L-cells
D. S-cells

123. A patient returns for a one-month follow-up visit with the dietician. Since the prior visit, the patient has not lost any weight and is frustrated, stating, "I can't lose any weight; I am a failure." Which of the following statements would most effectively assist with weight loss at his next visit?

A. What amount of weight loss would make you feel like you are successful?
B. I know it is frustrating, but I believe in you.
C. Have you been monitoring your caloric intake?
D. What is one thing you can change over the next month?

124. A weight management clinic acquires a duel-energy x-ray absorptiometry (DXA) scan that detects body mass which excludes both essential and nonessential fat. Which of the following terms does this describe?

A. Lean mass
B. Fat-free mass
C. Total body mass
D. Percent body fat

125. A local gym provides screening for cardiovascular risk factors and then provides a customized fitness plan to improve metabolic parameters. In particular, they focus on those with a moderate BMI with abdominal obesity. Which of the following ethnicities and waist circumferences would meet this parameter?

A. Caucasian male: 39 inches (99 cm)
B. Asian male: 31.5 inches (80 cm)
C. Caucasian female: 33 inches (83.3 cm)
D. Asian female: 35 inches (89 cm)

126. A 36-year-old female with type II diabetes wants to discuss different dietary patterns. She has a friend that had success with a ketogenic diet, and she was planning to initiate that eating plan on her return from vacation. Which of her medications should be discontinued before starting this diet?

A. Metformin
B. Insulin glargine
C. Dulaglutide
D. Empagliflozin

127. A 44-year-old male with a history of a recent duodenal switch presents to the emergency department with vomiting and ataxia. If this vitamin deficiency is not corrected, which of the following may be the clinical outcome?

A. Osteoporosis
B. Cardiomyopathy
C. Mucosal bleeding
D. Severe diarrhea

128. Which of the following is the best example of a SMART goal?

A. Lose weight by the end of the month by walking daily
B. Continue to avoid soda intake for the year
C. Reduce eating fast food to only once weekly
D. Hire a trainer to develop a weekly exercise plan

129. A 42-year-old male with class II obesity presents to the clinic for abnormalities on laboratory examination of the liver. In particular, his AST and ALT are elevated. He denies alcohol use. A liver biopsy is completed and shows hepatosteatitis. Which of the following is consistent with this diagnosis?

A. Fatty liver with the absence of inflammation
B. Hepatic injury present with irreversible nodules
C. Potential improvement from metformin use
D. Hepatic inflammation without cirrhosis

130. An asymptomatic patient undergoes a sleep study before bariatric surgery. During the study, she averaged ten episodes per 1 hour of oxygen desaturation from 98% to 93%, accompanied by periods of shallow breathing. Which finding does this most likely represent?

A. Apnea
B. Obstructive sleep apnea
C. Central sleep apnea
D. Hypopnea

131. Which of the following supplements is most closely associated with hepatic injury?

A. Green tea extract
B. Chitosan
C. Raspberry extract
D. Ephedra

132. A pediatric male patient presents to an obesity specialist to be evaluated for secondary causes of obesity. He has a history of seizures and developmental delay. On exam, he is noted to have more prominent earlobes and gynecomastia with underdeveloped genitals. What is the most likely syndrome?

A. Borgeson-Forssman-Lehmann
B. Cohen
C. Prader-Willi
D. Bardet-Biedl

133. The highest predictor of childhood obesity is in infants with which of the following characteristics?

A. Born one week past the due date
B. On-demand breast-fed infants
C. Marijuana use during pregnancy
D. Both parents have BMI ≥35 kg/m^2

134. A patient reads about a home remedy for weight loss that includes high doses of psyllium. The patient tolerates it initially but states it is causing gastrointestinal distress. Which mechanism is best attributed to her weight loss treatment?

A. Increased energy expenditure
B. Decreased dietary fat absorption
C. Increased fat oxidation
D. Improved satiety

135. A 17-year-old female underwent a Roux-en-Y gastric bypass. Twenty-four hours postoperatively, she complains of increasing abdominal and chest pain. The heart rate is elevated and blood counts reveal an elevated leukocyte count. Which of the following is the most likely cause of this patient's primary pathology causing her symptoms?

A. Pulmonary arteries
B. Pulmonary parenchyma
C. Gastrointestinal anastomosis site
D. Peritoneal and diaphragmatic surfaces

136. A study is being performed to determine the prevalence of vitamin deficiencies in those with obesity. One hundred participants undergo vitamin laboratory analysis. Which is the most prevalent deficiency in this population?

A. Thiamine
B. Iron
C. Vitamin D
D. Folate

137. A 9-year-old female presents with her parents to a pediatric weight management clinic. The patient's height, weight, and BMI have increased significantly over the past few years. The patient has developed breast buds. Which of the following is the most likely etiology?

A. Normal prepubertal development
B. Hypothyroidism
C. Increased caloric intake
D. Underlying genetic condition

138. Which of the following best describes the anatomical differences between a duodenal switch (DS) and a Roux-en-Y gastric bypass (RYGB)?

A. DS has a shorter common channel
B. RYGB removes a more significant portion of the stomach
C. The biliopancreatic loop in RYGB is primarily made from the jejunum
D. The digestive loop in the DS is most prone to small bacterial intestinal overgrowth

139. A patient was diagnosed with night eating syndrome and underwent cognitive behavioral therapy. Although improvements are noted in eating behaviors, the patient is interested in pharmacotherapy. Which of the following is the most efficacious option?

A. Phentermine
B. Metformin
C. Sertraline
D. Bupropion

140. A 26-year-old female presents for a gynecologic evaluation after being evaluated in the emergency department for pelvic pain. A pregnancy test was negative and an ultrasound revealed multiple bilateral ovarian cysts. Which of the following would most likely be decreased in this patient?

A. Sex hormone binding globulin
B. Luteinizing: follicular stimulating hormone ratio
C. Androgens
D. Prolactin

141. A female patient with pre-diabetes presents to her primary care physician to discuss the initiation of metformin. According to the American Diabetes Association, in what scenario should metformin be considered for this patient?

A. Age greater than 45 years old
B. History of gestational diabetes
C. A body mass index of 30 kg/m^2
D. A strong family history of diabetes

142. An exercise prescription is written for a patient following an initial consultation with an obesity medicine specialist. Regarding the acronym 'FITTE' used to write the script, what does the 'I' stand for?

A. Instructions
B. Intervals
C. Interests
D. Intensity

143. A psychiatrist meets with a patient for a consultation before a sleeve gastrectomy. She utilizes 'evoking,' a key process of motivational interviewing. What phrase is most consistent with that key process?

A. What is your most significant motivation to improve your health?
B. I want you to know that everything you tell me today is confidential.
C. Let's write out some short-term and long-term weight goals.
D. It seems like you struggle to eat healthily while at work. Tell me more about this.

144. Which would be a beneficial reason for allowing a pre-operative gastric bypass patient to consume carbohydrates up to 2 hours before anesthesia induction?

    A. Prevent post-operative nausea
    B. Allow for earlier detection of extraluminal leaks
    C. Improve insulin resistance
    D. Reduce the need for diphenoxylate postoperatively

145. Which of the following pediatric patients should start the 4-tiered approach for managing pediatric obesity, compared to those who can continue with prevention of obesity management only?

    A. A patient with a BMI in the 80th percentile with type 1 diabetes
    B. A patient with a BMI in the 85th percentile with tonsillar hypertrophy
    C. A patient with a BMI in the 90th percentile with Bartter syndrome
    D. A patient with a BMI in the 95th percentile with no comorbidities

146. The American College of Cardiology recommends which individuals undergo a stress electrocardiogram test if planning to start a vigorous exercise plan?

    A. Women > 50 years old who are asymptomatic
    B. Anyone over the age of 55 years with diabetes
    C. Deconditioned males over the age of 35 years old
    D. In those with a family history of cardiomyopathy

147. A clinic has created a limited program to capture and work closely with those at risk for obesity-related complications. This will include follow-up with a dietician and a trainer to provide a customized plan. Initially, they want to limit this to patients with a BMI of $\geq$ 30 kg/m^2. Of these patients, which ones should receive priority?

    A. Males with a waist circumference of 99 cm (39 inches)
    B. Patients with an Edmonton Obesity Staging System stage 2
    C. Patients with prediabetes or mild osteoarthritis
    D. Those with a family history of coronary artery disease

148. A 14-year-old male presents to clinic. His body mass index of 36 kg/m^2 is in the 99th percentile range based on age and gender. Which of the following most accurately describes his weight categorization?

A. Overweight
B. Obesity class I
C. Obesity class II
D. Obesity class III

149. The Centers for Disease Control and Prevention recognizes which of the following malignancies has a direct correlation with excess weight?

A. Testicular cancer
B. Colorectal cancer
C. Cholangiocarcinoma
D. Chronic Leukemia

150. A 54-year-old patient is admitted to the hospital with an elevated D-lactose level in the setting of encephalopathy and ataxia. The patient underwent a successful Roux-en-Y gastric bypass three years prior. Which of the following likely explains these findings?

A. Acute alcohol intoxication
B. Small intestinal bowel overgrowth
C. Thiamine deficiency
D. A surgical emergency

Practice Test 4

151. A pregnant female presents to her obstetrician and requests recommendations to ensure her infant doesn't develop obesity. She has struggled with weight throughout her adult life and wants to ensure her newborn has the best chance to maintain good health. What advice is most appropriate at this time?

A. Feed the infant a lower protein diet
B. Reduce carbohydrate-rich foods during pregnancy
C. Avoid breastfeeding the infant due to the high sugar content
D. Early complimentary feedings in an infant reduce the risk of obesity

152. A 51-year-old has neuropathy due to amyloidosis, as well as sleep-onset insomnia. The patient's BMI is 36 kg/m^2. Which medication would be most appropriate to start at this time?

A. Amitriptyline
B. Imipramine
C. Nortriptyline
D. Mirtazepine

153. A 33-year-old male presents for his 4-month post-Roux-en-Y gastric bypass surgery follow-up visit. He has not tolerated a solid diet and has been non-adherent with his medications. He is complaining of diarrhea which has not improved despite loperamide. On physical examination, a rash is noted on his lower extremities. Which finding would most likely occur if this particular vitamin deficiency is not corrected?

A. Memory issues
B. Lower extremity edema
C. Macrocytic anemia
D. Neuropathy

154. Which of the following is included in the diagnosis of metabolic syndrome?

A. Liver function tests
B. Low-density lipoprotein
C. Body mass index
D. Fasting plasma glucose

155. An elderly male with class I obesity is seen by a nursing home physician after being hospitalized for four weeks with COVID pneumonia. He does not have the strength to stand for longer than 1 minute and cannot perform repetitive tasks like raising his hands. His weight is now similar to his pre-covid diagnosis. What diagnosis most accurately reflects his findings?

A. Steroid-induced polymyositis
B. Sarcopenic obesity
C. Normal changes with aging
D. Malnourishment

156. Which of the following anorexigenic intestinal hormones is secreted by the small intestines to slow gastric emptying and aids in fat digestion?

A. Peptide YY
B. Glucagon-like peptide 1
C. Oxyntomodulin
D. Cholecystokinin

157. The OARS framework is utilized when performing motivational interviewing on a patient attempting to lose weight. What does the "O" stand for in this acronym?

A. Outside influences
B. Obstructions that require a change
C. Open-ended questions
D. Opportunities to change

158. A 63-year-old male presents to a metabolic and bariatric surgical clinic to discuss weight loss options. He has read about the TransPyloric Shuttle® and would like to know if he is a candidate for this device placement. Which of the following is a contraindication to this device?

A. History of colectomy due to colon cancer
B. Taking anticoagulation for atrial fibrillation
C. Treatment for H. Pylori within the past six months
D. Prior history of NSAID-induced gastric ulcer

159. A patient underwent the most common bariatric surgery and is doing well afterward. Which of the following is most likely decreased in this patient post-operatively?

A. Cells directly producing ghrelin
B. Risk of acid reflux
C. Glucagon-like peptide 1 secretion
D. Vitamin absorptive capacity

160. The federal government approves a graduated budgetary allowance to the states with the highest rates of obesity prevalence. Which state would likely receive the most significant financial influx?

A. California
B. Colorado
C. West Virginia
D. Florida

161. A maximum dose of phentermine/topiramate ER (Qsymia®) would include what dose range for the topiramate ER?

A. 0-25 mg
B. 25-50 mg
C. 50-75 mg
D. 75-100 mg

162. A patient saw the term "adiposopathy" on their chart and was unsure how this related to her comorbidities of obesity. Which of the following conditions is this likely referring to?

A. Atherosclerosis of the carotid artery
B. Heart failure with a preserved ejection fraction
C. Osteoarthritis of the knees
D. Obstructive sleep apnea

163. A 33-year-old female would like to undergo bariatric surgery to improve her health and reduce her risk of future pregnancy complications. She has been diagnosed with polycystic ovarian syndrome, which has impaired her ability to become pregnant. She is hoping that with substantial weight loss, she will be more likely to become pregnant. What is the minimum recommended time frame after surgery she should be instructed to avoid pregnancy?

    A. 3 months
    B. 6 months
    C. 9 months
    D. 12 months

164. A patient undergoes a dual-energy x-ray absorptiometry test to determine his body fat percentage. Which of the following best reflects this testing modality?

    A. It is considered the gold standard
    B. Any BMI can undergo this testing
    C. It is associated with significant radiation exposure
    D. It is inaccurate if the patient is dehydrated

165. A 12-year-old male presents to his pediatrician with an abnormal gait. His parents have noticed it more during the pandemic when they state his weight has increased due to less physical activity. Examination reveals bowing of the tibia. His mother states there are no dietary restrictions. Which of the following is the most likely etiology of his presentation?

    A. Ricket's
    B. Legg-Calve-Perthes disease
    C. Slipped capital femoral epiphysis
    D. Blount disease

166. A 39-year-old female presents to a family medicine physician frustrated by her inability to lose weight over the past six months. Despite increased exercise and improved eating habits, she feels more tired and gained approximately 15 lbs (6.8kg) over the same time frame. Which skin finding would most likely be seen on physical exam?

    A. Widened abdominal striae
    B. Xanthelasmas
    C. Acne
    D. Dry and cracked skin

167. Where is the location of vitamin B_{12} absorption within the gastrointestinal tract?

    A. Gastric fundus
    B. Proximal small intestines
    C. Distal small intestines
    D. Colon

168. The consequences of maternal obesity and the intrauterine environment in which a fetus develops affect which of the following?

    A. Genetic mutations
    B. Mitochondrial deletions
    C. DNA expression
    D. Recessive inheritance

169. Out of 1000 kcal utilized throughout a day in a resting individual, how many calories would the skeletal muscles consume?

    A. 50 kcal
    B. 100 kcal
    C. 150 kcal
    D. 200 kcal

170. A 61-year-old female who underwent a biliopancreatic diversion with duodenal switch six years prior returns for her annual follow-up appointment. She underwent a dual-energy x-ray absorptiometry and was found to have a T score of -2.6 (reference range: between +1 and -1). She had normal vitamin levels and an unremarkable complete metabolic panel. Which of the following is recommended at this time?

A. Weekly oral alendronate
B. Daily oral alendronate
C. Intravenous zoledronic acid annually
D. One-time subcutaneous denosumab injection

171. In those 2-19 years old, who has the highest prevalence rates of obesity?

A. Those with the highest income
B. Caucasian females
C. Asian males
D. Middle-income families

172. A local supermarket is advertising a new dietary supplement they just started selling. Which of the following describes this substance most accurately?

A. It is considered safe according to the FDA
B. It can be marketed to prevent but not cure diseases
C. It is considered a food, not a drug
D. It has positive effects beyond basic nutrition

173. A 51-year-old female presents to clinic for smoking cessation and is prescribed bupropion. Five days later, she is brought to the emergency department by ambulance with convulsive seizures. Which of the following was likely not addressed at the time of medication initiation?

A. Concurrent marijuana use
B. Parotid gland enlargement on exam
C. Current prescription of sertraline
D. Family history of a cranial neoplasm

174. An 18-year-old returns from college after her first semester. Her body mass index (BMI) 6 months ago was 29 kg/m². However, with her lack of physical activity and increased caloric intake, her BMI has now increased by 2 kg/m². Which of the following would best classify her new BMI?

A. Normal weight
B. Overweight
C. Class I obesity
D. Class II obesity

175. Two adolescent patients are seen in a tertiary weight management facility. One has a leptin receptor gene defect and the other has melanocortin 4 receptor deficiency. What will be the most noticeable difference between these two patients?

A. Height
B. Skin pallor
C. Blood pressure
D. Intellectual ability

176. The mechanism and effect behind dumping syndrome after a patient undergoes a Roux-en-Y gastric bypass is best described by which of the following statements?

A. High protein osmotic gradient causes rapid gut transit time
B. Exaggerated insulin secretion leads to hypoglycemia
C. Large carbohydrate loads cause increased bacterial gas production
D. The bypassed pylorus is unable to regulate the rate of acidotic gastric contents

177. During an evaluation for weight loss surgery, a dietician estimates the patient's total energy expenditure (TEE). The dietician tells the patient the TEE may be under-evaluated due to non-exercise activity thermogenesis. What is the dietician referring to?

A. Calories utilized while sleeping
B. Energy utilized to digest foods
C. Walking with her spouse in the evenings
D. Energy expended while tapping her foot

178. A 43-year-old female presents with worsening acne over the past year. She has gained some weight, although she feels it has mostly accumulated in her abdomen. Which of the following tests is most appropriate at this time?

A. DHEA-S
B. MRI of the pituitary
C. Buccal salivary swab
D. Cosyntropin stimulation test

179. A 39-year-old female presents to clinic with persistent symptoms of feeling flushed, lightheaded, and mild confusion. She underwent a sleeve gastrectomy one year prior but noted symptoms even before surgery. She is otherwise healthy, although she underwent a parathyroidectomy three months prior with recent electrolytes within normal limits. Which of the following is most likely associated with her findings?

A. Elevated fasting c-peptide
B. Female predominance of this disorder
C. Symptom improvement with increased protein intake
D. Normal fasting glucose with post-prandial hypoglycemia

180. A 29-year-old male presents to an urgent care for COVID symptoms. He states that although he has no respiratory symptoms, his taste seems abnormal. He says it is particularly noticeable when drinking soda. His rapid COVID test is negative. Upon medication review, which of the following is most likely the culprit for his current symptoms?

A. Bupropion
B. Semaglutide
C. Topiramate
D. Phentermine

181. A 29-year-old female has been working vigorously over the past six months to increase her fitness level and decrease her weight before her upcoming wedding. After the wedding, she reduced her exercise routine to three times weekly and is frustrated she is starting to regain weight. Which of the following is likely to blame for her recent weight gain?

A. Adaptive thermogenesis
B. Commitment amnesia
C. Neurohurmonal influences
D. Increased muscle efficiency

182. A patient immediately after a Roux-en-Y surgery is difficult to extubate and eventually requires reintubation while still in the postanesthesia unit. A chest x-ray is normal, a complete blood count is normal, and a metabolic panel shows decreased bicarbonate. What is the most likely diagnosis?

A. Anastomotic leak
B. Pulmonary embolism
C. Obstructive sleep apnea
D. Pseudocholinesterase deficiency

183. Statistics are being evaluated to determine how income and education levels affect rates of obesity in adults. Which of the following would be expected to have the highest rates of obesity?

A. Well-educated females
B. Men living in poverty
C. Men in the middle class
D. Females in the middle class

184. Which of the following should be available in all physician's offices that treat patients with obesity?

A. Exam tables that can accommodate 300 lbs
B. Open scales available in public areas
C. Chairs without side rails
D. Sheets to cover the patients instead of gowns

185. Which pediatric condition is associated with enlarged organs and hepatoblastoma?

A. Cohen syndrome
B. Alstrom syndrome
C. Beckwith-Wiedemann syndrome
D. Prader-Willi syndrome

186. A metabolic and bariatric surgery center is evaluating a 44-year-old female. During the initial consult, she admits to eating until uncomfortably full and feeling guilty afterward. Although she states some of the guilt has caused her to seek bariatric surgery options, she denies any excessive exercise or dietary changes. What other item is she most likely to admit to?

A. Hiding her eating behaviors
B. Waking up in the night to eat
C. Consuming most of her calories at night
D. Induced vomiting after meals

187. A child has received a diagnosis of proopiomelanocortin deficiency. A melanocortin 4 receptor agonist will be initiated. Which other condition is this medication indicated?

    A. Leptin receptor deficiency
    B. Prader-Willi syndrome
    C. Class III pediatric obesity
    D. Alstrom syndrome

188. What is the relationship between fat-free mass and lean body mass?

    A. Lean body mass and fat-free mass are within 15-20% of each other
    B. Lean body mass includes fat in the bone marrow and central nervous system
    C. Fat-free mass excludes nonessential fat but includes essential fat
    D. These terms are theoretical and not able to be detected on imaging

189. Immediately before bariatric surgery, the patient should do which of the following?

    A. Take oral nonsteroidal anti-inflammatories
    B. Perform deep breathing exercises
    C. Start pharmacologic deep venous thrombosis prophylaxis
    D. Be administered approximately 2 liters of lactated ringers

190. A patient eats six servings of fruit per day. How many total calories does this add to his daily caloric intake?

    A. 180 calories
    B. 240 calories
    C. 360 calories
    D. 420 calories

191. Which of the following patients who have failed lifestyle modifications meet the criteria for anti-obesity medications?

A. A patient with a BMI of 26 kg/m² who has a strong family history of obesity
B. A patient with a BMI of 28 kg/m² who has polycystic ovarian syndrome
C. A patient with a BMI of 29 kg/m² on pitavastatin
D. A patient with a BMI of 30 kg/m² who is a bodybuilder

192. A 26-year-old female presents to the dietician for an initial consult for weight management. She has a history of obstructive sleep apnea and recurrent abdominal intertrigo. She inquires about the most effective dietary plan. What is the best response?

A. Adherence to a dietary plan long-term is required to be successful
B. The Mediterranean diet is anti-inflammatory and would help with the intertrigo
C. Strict low carbohydrates would be preferred to help with initial rapid weight loss
D. Calorie restriction to 1500 kcal/day provides a consistent calorie deficit

193. A patient undergoing weight management with naltrexone/bupropion ER admits to relapsing with intravenous heroin. Her urine drug screen is positive for heroin and hydrocodone. She admits her last dose of heroin was last night, and she took hydrocodone this morning. Which of the following recommendation should be provided?

A. Stop your naltrexone/bupropion ER immediately
B. Change to naltrexone monotherapy, as it can be used to treat opioid use disorder
C. Decrease opioid use while discontinuing the anti-obesity medication
D. Change to bupropion ER monotherapy for continued weight benefits

194. At what minimum glomerular filtration rate are all FDA-approved long-term weight loss medications safe to use without a restriction in dosing?

A. 15 mL/min
B. 30 mL/min
C. 45 mL/min
D. 60 mL/min

195. A patient presents to her family practitioner for general health counseling. Which of the following would be consistent with tertiary prevention?

A. Education on the prevention of obesity
B. Initiate lifestyle interventions to decrease weight
C. Start pharmacotherapy to prevent weight-related complications
D. Initiate semaglutide to improve diabetes control

196. A patient who successfully underwent bariatric surgery has been losing weight steadily. Which of the following should be recommended to this patient?

A. Continue your current dietary and physical activity plan until you are at your goal weight
B. Intensify your exercise regimen as you continue to lose weight
C. Adjust caloric intake by 50 calories/day until consistently losing weight
D. Continue a liquid diet until at target weight, then introduce solids

197. A 41-year-old patient, who was started on liraglutide two months prior for weight loss, is admitted to the emergency department with severe right-sided flank pain and hematuria. A renal stone passes the following day spontaneously. What is the most likely mechanism liraglutide contributed to her presentation?

A. Rapid weight loss
B. Volume contraction
C. Increased oxalate absorption
D. Reduced calcium excretion

198. What is the minimal Tanner Stage required in an adolescent to meet metabolic and bariatric surgery criteria?

    A. Tanner Stage 1
    B. Tanner Stage 2
    C. Tanner Stage 3
    D. Tanner Stage 4

199. What term best describes when a victim becomes the target of unfavorable treatment?

    A. Stigma
    B. Prejudice
    C. Harassment
    D. Bias

200. A 17-year-old female presents with migraines and excess weight. She is interested in starting topiramate, as her mother had improvements with this medication. The patient is sexually active, uses condoms occasionally, and refuses to use birth control regularly. The physician refuses to prescribe topiramate. What ethical principle is involved in this decision?

    A. Justice
    B. Nonmaleficence
    C. Autonomy
    D. Beneficence

Practice Test 5

201. A patient plans to undergo metabolic and bariatric surgery within the next three months. If found upon endoscopy, which of the following should a Roux-en-Y gastric bypass be recommended over a sleeve gastrectomy?

    A. Intestinal metaplasia in the esophagus
    B. Gastric food remnants despite being NPO for 12 hours
    C. Helical-shaped, gram-negative bacteria in the stomach
    D. Visible scarring from a previous PEG tube

202. A 7-year-old male is sent to an endocrinologist due to abnormal electrolytes, including hypocalcemia and hyperphosphatemia. He has round facies, a high body mass index, and shorter stature. Which of the following conditions is most associated with these findings?

    A. Albright-Hereditary Osteodystrophy
    B. Prader-Willi syndrome
    C. Proopiomelanocortin gene mutation
    D. Bardet-Biedl syndrome

203. A patient presents for a metabolic surgery screening consultation with an obesity medicine specialist. She does have slight hirsutism and admits to irregular periods. She also has striae on her abdomen. She has not been in a structured weight program previously. Which of the following should be recommended at this time?

    A. Minimum weight loss of 15 lbs (6.8 kg) before surgery
    B. Testing for sex hormonal abnormalities
    C. Overnight dexamethasone suppression test
    D. Six months of a structured weight loss program

204. An endoscopically placed weight loss device that can remain in place for one year, and works by helping delay the gastric transit of food content, describes which of the following?

    A. Aspiration device
    B. Intragastric balloon
    C. TransPyloric Shuttle
    D. Sleeve gastroplasty

205. A male patient presents to his primary care physician complaining of excessive burping. Recently, he started supplements to help with weight loss. Which of the following supplements is most likely contributing to his presentation?

A. Glucosinolates
B. Green tea extract
C. Raspberry ketones
D. Chitosan

206. The maximum dose of bupropion in the combination anti-obesity medication Naltrexone/bupropion ER (Contrave®) is between what values?

A. 0-100 mg/day
B. 100-200 mg/day
C. 200-300 mg/day
D. 300-400 mg/day

207. A patient is interested in starting semaglutide (Wegovy®). The maximum weekly dose, if tolerated, is between which of the following ranges?

A. 0.5 to 1 mg
B. 1 to 1.5 mg
C. 1.5 to 2 mg
D. 2 to 2.5 mg

208. Appropriate testosterone replacement in a male with hypogonadism is most likely to improve which of the following conditions?

A. Blood pressure
B. Lipid panel
C. Sleep apnea
D. Fertility

209. A recently married male presents for discussion of increased weight gain. He states since moving in with his wife, he feels more fatigued and hungrier throughout the daytime. He goes to bed and wakes up at similar times compared to before marriage. He was tested for sleep apnea one year ago, which was negative. What other question may help to determine his increased appetite?

A. Have you had recent thyroid studies?
B. Does your wife have restless leg syndrome?
C. Do you take melatonin before bedtime?
D. Was the sleep study done in a sleep center or at home?

210. Which class of medications used for diabetes prevents the breakdown of the incretins glucagon-like peptide 1 and gastric inhibitory peptide, increasing pancreatic insulin synthesis and decreasing glucagon?

A. DDP-4 inhibitors
B. SGLT2- inhibitors
C. Metformin
D. Sulfonylureas

211. The principle of "doing what is best for the patient" falls under which ethical principle?

A. Justice
B. Nonmaleficence
C. Autonomy
D. Beneficence

212. "Perform 45 minutes of water walking at 2 miles per hour every Monday, Wednesday, and Friday before work. In addition, lift weights for 15 minutes on days that you do not swim." This statement describes which of the following?

A. A SMART goal
B. An exercise prescription
C. 'Arrange/Assist' component of the 5 A's of obesity management
D. Component of motivational interviewing

213. A male presents to an obesity medicine clinic as he was told that he was considered to have obesity based on his percentage of fat. Which of the following is the minimum percentage of body fat to meet this criterion in this patient?

  A. 23%
  B. 28%
  C. 32%
  D. 38%

214. A 15-year-old female who underwent a sleeve gastrectomy nine months prior is returning due to increasing weight over the prior two months. Although she no longer runs outside due to the cold winter, she has maintained 300 mins/week of moderate physical activity at the gym. She denies other stressors. Which of the following should be recommended at this time?

  A. Strict documentation of calorie intake
  B. Increasing physical activity by 20%
  C. Surgery re-evaluation for potential anatomic etiology
  D. Laboratory assessment

215. A 6-year-old male patient presents to the pediatrician for recurrent shoulder dislocations. His joints are hypermobile. He is minimally interactive and does not make eye contact but has an open-mouth expression. His vision is poor. He has thickened hair and eyebrows. This condition is characterized by what genetic abnormality?

  A. Autosomal dominant
  B. Autosomal recessive
  C. X-linked recessive
  D. X-linked dominant

216. A 26-year-old male, not on any medications, has a diagnosis of metabolic syndrome according to the National Cholesterol Education Program (NCEP) Adult Treatment Panel III (ATP III). Which of the following characteristics is likely to be present in this patient?

A. Triglycerides of 140 mg/dL (reference range < 150 mg/dL)
B. HbA1c of 6.1% (reference range < 5.7%)
C. Total cholesterol of 210 mg/dL (reference range <200 mg/dL)
D. Blood pressure of 128/80 mmHg

217. An 11-year-old female is diagnosed with new-onset hypertension and prediabetes. Upon further workup, an adrenal adenoma secreting excess cortisol is discovered. Which of the following growth chart characteristics is likely seen in this patient?

A. Proportional weight and height increases
B. Increased height compared to weight
C. Normal growth charts
D. Increased weight compared to height

218. Exogenous leptin is injected into a test subject. This hormone is found to stimulate which of the following pathways?

A. Cocaine and amphetamine-regulated transcript
B. Neuropeptide Y
C. Agouti-related peptide
D. Y1 and Y5 receptors

219. A patient is asked a series of questions about the likelihood of falling asleep during certain activities throughout the day. These questions are screening for a condition directly associated with which of the following parameters?

A. Elevated FVC/FEV$_1$ ratio
B. Increased respiratory disturbance index
C. Elevated daytime carbon dioxide
D. Prolonged QRS interval

220. A patient starts taking a daily pill that she states is advertised to help stimulate healthy intestinal bacterial growth, which promotes a microbiome conducive to weight loss. Which of the following does this describe?

A. Dietary fiber
B. Oligosaccharides
C. Probiotics
D. Stool softener

221. Which of the following statements is true regarding the use of warfarin in patients who have undergone bariatric surgery and developed postoperative venous thromboembolism (VTE)?

A. Warfarin is preferred because it can be monitored closely
B. Warfarin should never be used after a gastric bypass
C. In the setting of an acute DVT, bridge warfarin with enoxaparin
D. Avoid using warfarin initially, but it is still an option

222. A 32-year-old male presents to the clinic to inquire about injectable weight loss medications. In particular, he is interested in one that is also used in diabetes. Which of the following may be a relative contraindication of this medication?

A. Pituitary adenoma
B. Calcitonin elevation
C. History of volvulus
D. Glaucoma

223. Patients with which of the following comorbidities should cellulose and citric acid be avoided?

A. Plummer Vinson syndrome
B. Gastrointestinal reflux disease
C. Celiac disease
D. Irritable bowel syndrome

224. An administrator is trying to determine the extra cost burden for employees that have the disease of obesity. He has categorized costs into indirect and direct. In this scenario, an example of indirect costs would include which of the following?

A. Absenteeism
B. Physician visits
C. Prescription drug use
D. Hospitalizations

225. A female is presenting for her three-month follow-up appointment. Over the past two years, she has successfully lost 45 lbs (20.4 kg). As the holidays are coming, she is fearful as she knows this is her most challenging time regarding excess eating due to the number of family events scheduled. Which of the following questions is most appropriate?

A. Given your weight loss, don't you feel like you deserve to reward yourself?
B. What is your goal weight after the holidays?
C. Are there any other family members going through a similar weight loss journey?
D. What could you eat before the event to curb your appetite?

226. A research study recruits 1,000 individuals with the disease of obesity. What is the highest prevalence gene most likely seen in this population?

A. LEPR
B. FTO
C. MC4R
D. POMC

227. The United States Department of Agriculture provides what acceptable macronutrient distribution range for fat intake?

A. 5-15%
B. 15-25%
C. 25-35%
D. 35-40%

228. A 14-year-old female, with the agreement of her parents, has decided to pursue a sleeve gastrectomy due to her persistently elevated body mass index, pre-diabetes, and obstructive sleep apnea. Which of the following would be a contraindication to surgery?

A. Heroin use 2 months ago
B. A BMI in the 125% of the 95th percentile
C. Tanner Stage 2
D. Alcohol use within the past month

229. A patient has a one-month follow-up visit for new-onset hypertension. He states he feels well and denies any new complaints. A review of records shows a body mass index (BMI) increase of 3 kg/m^2 over the past month without an increase in waist circumference. Persistent trace edema is present. Which of the following conditions likely led to his increased BMI?

A. Nephrotic syndrome
B. Vertebral compression fracture
C. Seasonal clothing changes
D. Increased dietary intake

230. A 66-year-old female has read about a new diet plan that restricts fruits but allows increased protein intake. She feels this would be a good fit, as she has a barbeque business. Which of the following is this dietary plan most similar to?

A. Dietary approach to stop hypertension (DASH)
B. Paleo diet
C. Carbohydrate restricted diet
D. Mediterranean diet

231. What is one of the potentially negative effects of oxyntomodulin?

A. Blockade of GLP-1 receptors
B. Increased risk of gallstones
C. Glucagon agonist
D. Hypoglycemic effects

232. A 24-year-old male is found deep within the woods. He states he wanted to go on a 3-month camping trip in which he secluded himself from the world and lived "off the land." He previously had minimal experience camping and stated he mostly consumed fish and occasional rabbits. He avoided berries or plants as he was unsure which were safe to eat. Which of the following is likely to be seen on physical examination?

A. Night blindness
B. Perifollicular hemorrhage
C. Anasarca
D. Koilonychia

233. The recommended daily caloric intake for females to obtain an energy deficit of at least 500 kcal/day is closest to which of the following?

A. 900 kcal/day
B. 1100 kcal/day
C. 1300 kcal/day
D. 1600 kcal/day

234. A patient status-post Roux-en-Y gastric bypass complains of lightheadedness and flushing after meals. In terms of timing, how could post-gastric bypass hypoglycemia (PGBH) and early dumping syndrome (DS) be differentiated?

A. DS occurs 1-4 hours after meals
B. PGBH is generally seen > 1 year after surgery
C. Symptoms of dumping syndrome last for > 30 minutes
D. PGBH symptoms can persist for > 4 hours

235. A patient presents for dietary follow-up. Although he has changed his eating habits to include more fruits, vegetables, and avoidance of soda, he has not appreciated much improvement in his weight. He is frustrated and states, "I will never lose weight. These changes were a waste of time." The dietician states, "You have already shown a lot of initiative in your lifestyle modifications. Let's see how we can channel that to other areas like physical activity." What motivational interview principle was displayed?

A. Empathy
B. Avoiding arguments
C. Resolving ambivalence
D. Developing discrepancy

236. A 27-year-old female with a BMI of 29 kg/m^2 presents for pre-conception counseling. Her smartwatch has been calculating approximately 5 hours of sleep nightly. What findings would be expected to increase if she improved her nightly sleep duration?

A. Ghrelin
B. Neuropeptide Y
C. Proopiomelanocortin
D. Melanin-concentrating hormone

237. A pathologist uses a special dye within the pancreas to identify prominent areas of hormone secretion. The stain for amylin would be seen within which cells?

A. Alpha cells
B. Beta cells
C. Delta cells
D. Gamma cells

238. A surgeon has collaborated with an anesthesiologist for pre-operative evaluation for patients planning to undergo metabolic and bariatric surgery. The assessment will be completed one week before the surgery date. Which of the following patients should have surgery delayed or canceled due to an elevated perioperative risk?

A. A patient over the age of 65 years old with sleep apnea
B. A patient who quit smoking cigarettes 3 months ago
C. A patient with factor 5 Leiden deficiency on apixaban
D. A female who stopped oral contraceptives 1 week ago

239. A 45-year-old male with a BMI of 62 kg/m^2 presents for a follow-up visit regarding his weight. Since his last visit, he has increased his water walking to 1 hour per day, four days during the week, and has maintained a 1600 kcal/day caloric intake. What would be the best advice to provide at this time?

A. Increase water walking to 5 days per week
B. Restrict calories an additional 400 kcal/day
C. Lift weights on weekends
D. Walk on the treadmill on days when not water walking

240. A patient is undergoing testing to determine their total energy expenditure (TEE). The value of energy expenditure from physical activity is estimated to be which approximate percentage of TEE?

A. 10%
B. 25%
C. 40%
D. 60%

241. A bodybuilder undergoes a program to improve strength and endurance. Measurements are taken throughout the 12-week course to see the progression. In particular, his percent body fat is measured. What formula best describes this measurement?

A. Total mass – fat mass
B. Fat mass/(total body mass – bone mass)
C. Total mass – fat mass – bone mineral content
D. Fat mass + lean mass + bone mass

242. During a lifestyle improvement lecture, a dietician recommends that a daily intake of 400 international units of vitamin D would be sufficient to meet the requirements of nearly all healthy, non-pregnant female patients. This amount of vitamin D meets the criteria for which of the following?

A. Daily value
B. Recommended dietary allowance
C. Estimated average requirement
D. Adequate intake

243. A mother asks her family practitioner how to assist her 11-year-old daughter in maintaining a healthy weight. During the COVID pandemic, the daughter reduced her physical activity and increased her caloric intake. This has led to increased weight. Which of the following is the best advice?

A. Encourage her to jog for 1 hour daily in the evening or morning
B. Allow the patient to eat more frequent smaller meals
C. Exchange one restaurant meal for a home-cooked family meal
D. Encourage her to reduce her time in front of her bedroom television

244. A 49-year-old patient with long-standing diabetes, controlled on metformin for the past seven years, presents for follow-up after being told she has "low blood counts" during a life-insurance screening exam. Given her medical history, what vitamin should be checked?

A. Iron
B. Folate
C. Cyanocobalamin
D. Copper

245. A weight management clinic is discussing options to determine metabolic rate. Which statement is most accurate regarding the relationship between resting metabolic rate (RMR) and basal metabolic rate (BMR)?

A. BMR is easier to obtain in an office setting
B. RMR requires an individual to be fasting
C. Total energy expenditure is based on BMR only
D. BMR and RMR are both increased with increased weight

246. A 19-year-old has recently started eating healthy and initiated a physical activity plan at his university this past month. He has never been in a program like this but is enjoying it, and he wants to be able to participate in intermural sports in the upcoming season. Which of the following would be important to help in his current goals at this stage?

A. Build awareness and discuss risks and benefits
B. Set goals and develop an action plan
C. Reward and encourage small changes
D. Discuss lapse and relapse coaching

247. A patient presents with peripheral edema, neuropathy, and a new S3 on physical examination. Upon further review, the patient has been consuming a severely calorie-deficient diet to lose weight over an extended period. Based on symptoms, what deficiency is likely present?

    A. Mineral
    B. Fat-soluble vitamin
    C. Total protein
    D. Water-soluble vitamin

248. The enhanced recovery after bariatric surgery (ERABS) recommendations include

    A. administering intra-operative regional blocks
    B. increasing tidal volume to maximally tolerated
    C. delaying post-operative oral intake until bowel function returns
    D. providing preoperative blood transfusion to improve hemodynamics

249. A 47-year-old male presents to his cardiologist for an annual evaluation. The prior year, he underwent a successful right coronary artery stent for stable coronary artery disease. Which anthropometric measurements would be the best predictor of future mortality?

    A. Waist circumference
    B. Body mass index
    C. Resting metabolic rate
    D. Skin fold calipers

250. The trend of Roux-en-Y gastric bypass (RYGB) over the past ten years is best described by which of the following sentences?

    A. The numbers of RYGB declined initially, followed by a steady incline.
    B. RYGB makes up approximately half of the bariatric surgeries.
    C. The percentage of RYGB is now similar to the percentage of bariatric revisions.
    D. The number of RYGB has continued to increase in the pediatric patient population.

Practice Test 6

251. Which patient characteristic would have a relatively higher lean body mass?

A. Male gender
B. Older individual
C. Sedentary individual
D. Patient with cachexia

252. A patient presents to the emergency department with persistent fatigue, loss of appetite, and anasarca. Labs reveal a high anion gap metabolic acidosis and renal failure. Which of the following medications most likely led to the acid-base disorder?

A. Metformin
B. Topiramate
C. Phentermine
D. Bupropion

253. A very motivated patient presents to the clinic in January after making a New Year's Resolution for weight loss. He wants to be aggressive with his approach and has researched a very low-calorie diet (VLCD). What is an appropriate statement about this approach?

A. It has been shown to have greater long-term weight effects
B. A VLCD tends to be more cost-effective
C. Complication risks are eliminated if monitored monthly
D. Patients on this diet intake significant amounts of protein

254. A 44-year-old female recently started on semaglutide for diabetes and concurrent weight loss. Which of the following parameters will likely increase as a result of starting this therapy?

A. HDL cholesterol
B. Triglycerides
C. Hemoglobin A1c
D. Diastolic blood pressure

255. A 39-year-old female presents with painful bumps that begin to develop over the thighs and abdomen. On examination, multiple discrete subcutaneous nodules are palpable, ranging in size from 3-6 mm. What is the most likely etiology of this finding?

A. Dercum's disease
B. Lipedema
C. Lymphedema
D. Lipodystrophy

256. A 45-year-old male with class II obesity presents to the emergency department in cardiac arrest. Family members state he went on an extreme diet, only drinking water for the past three weeks. He had lost a significant amount of weight but became weak and irritable, per the family. Today he decided to break his fast by ordering a pizza. Shortly after his meal, he became unconscious, and an ambulance was called. What deficiency most likely lead to his current condition?

A. Phosphate
B. Thiamine
C. Calcium
D. Potassium

257. A 49-year-old female with a history of type II diabetes presents to her primary care clinician to discuss her recent lab work. She is currently on metformin and her most recent hemoglobin A1c was 9.1% (reference range < 5.7%). She is planning to start a ketogenic diet to help with diabetes control but is also open to starting a new medication. Which of the following classes of medications should be avoided at this time?

A. GLP-1 receptor agonist
B. DPP4 inhibitor
C. SGLT-2 inhibitor
D. Thiazolidinedione

258. In calculating the resting energy expenditure, which of the following components plays the most prominent role in the Mifflin St. Jeor equation equation?

    A. Age
    B. Gender
    C. Weight
    D. Height

259. A young child was recently diagnosed with Angelman syndrome. What is the genetic etiology of this condition?

    A. Autosomal recessive
    B. Maternal imprinting error
    C. Paternal deletion of 15q13
    D. Trisomy

260. A 29-year-old female presents to her obstetrician for her 20-week fetal ultrasound evaluation. She became pregnant two months after a Roux-en-Y gastric bypass and takes bariatric vitamins sporadically. During the exam, a fetal abnormality is noted on the midline of the spine. Intake of which of the following vitamins would have prevented this complication?

    A. Folate
    B. Cyanocobalamin
    C. Thiamine
    D. Copper

261. A study is being conducted to determine the differences in hormone levels in men versus women at equivalent body mass index values. It will likely be found that compared to women, men have

    A. higher levels of adiponectin
    B. lower levels of leptin
    C. equivalent sex hormone binding globulin levels
    D. decreased lean body mass

262. A 20-year-old female presents to discuss exercise recommendations. She is planning to perform 300 minutes of moderate-intensity exercise weekly. She would like to target a specific heart rate to determine her level of physical intensity. What is the recommended heart rate to target for moderate-intensity exercise?

A. 100 BPM (50% of max predicted heart rate)
B. 120 BPM (60% of max predicted heart rate)
C. 140 BPM (70% of max predicted heart rate)
D. 160 BPM (80% of max predicted heart rate)

263. Which of the following medications used for diabetes is considered weight-neutral?

A. Metformin
B. Sitagliptin
C. Exenatide
D. Glipizide

264. What inheritance pattern is Wilson-Turner syndrome?

A. Autosomal dominant
B. Autosomal recessive
C. X-Linked
D. Trisomy

265. A study utilizing a functional MRI is being conducted. Images of food are displayed to the research participant while they are in an MRI. The researcher can visualize activated areas within the brain in real time. One particular image activates the amygdala. Which of the following qualities about the food image likely caused this activation?

A. A memory associated with the image
B. A prior food addiction
C. Ghrelin stimulation of NPY/AgRP
D. A successful advertisement

266. A study comparing the relative risk of mortality between those with a normal BMI and those with a BMI ≥ 40 kg/m^2 is most likely to discover that females with higher BMIs have a greater relative risk of which cancer?

A. Colon
B. Endometrial
C. Pancreatic
D. Breast

267. Which of the following patients is most likely to have a higher VO$_2$ max?

A. A 23-year-old male who swims 30 minutes daily
B. A 65-year-old female who walks 2 miles daily
C. A 50-year-old male with a body fat percentage of 36%
D. A 33-year-old male with Down syndrome

268. A 68-year-old male with class II obesity underwent a heart catheterization after having a stress test showing reversible myocardial ischemia. He is started on aspirin and clopidogrel. The cardiologist asks you to start a beta-blocker. Which of the following is the most appropriate medication to start?

A. Carvedilol
B. Metoprolol succinate
C. Atenolol
D. Metoprolol tartrate

269. A 12-year-old male is being treated for a genetic cause of obesity. The medication has worked well, but the child admits to having spontaneous erections that have become bothersome. Which of the following medications is he most likely taking?

A. Metreleptin
B. Setmelanotide
C. Semaglutide
D. Tirzepatide

270. A 56-year-old female underwent a sleeve gastrectomy two years prior and has lost nearly 100 lbs (45.5 kg) since surgery. She feels tired, wakes up with night sweats, and continues to lose weight. She has a decreased appetite but denies stomach pains. She continues to lose weight and is now in the underweight category. All vitamin and laboratory work is normal. What is the most likely etiology of her symptoms?

A. Menopause
B. Underlying malignancy
C. Dumping syndrome
D. Depression

271. A patient intakes 10 grams of carbohydrates. How many kcal did they consume?

A. 20 kcal
B. 40 kcal
C. 70 kcal
D. 90 kcal

272. A 21-year-old female patient is discussing weight during pre-conception counseling. She has a strong family history of obesity, although she and her husband have normal body mass indexes. Which of the following could contribute to the risk of obesity in her children later in life?

A. Exclusively breastfeeding for the first six months
B. Physical abuse in the household
C. Education within a private school setting
D. Vaginal delivery causing a perineal laceration

273. A 39-year-old male presents to the clinic for headaches. He has a history of hypogonadism treated with intramuscular testosterone and obstructive sleep apnea treated with continuous positive airway pressure. He underwent a sleeve gastrectomy the year prior and lost 62 lbs (28.1 kg). Labs reveal a hemoglobin level of 19.3 g/dL (reference range: 13.5–17.5 g/dL) with a low erythropoietin level. What is the most important next step?

A. Obtain a renal ultrasound
B. Repeat levels in 1 month
C. Reduce the testosterone dose
D. Repeat a sleep study

274. A physician is seeing a patient in the bariatric clinic. The patient states that "weight loss is as simple as calories in and calories out." The physician resists the desire to correct him but instead tries to understand where the patient is coming from. This motivational technique is best described by which of the following models?

A. OARS
B. RULE
C. FRAMES
D. PACE

275. A 21-year-old male begins complaining of significant abdominal pain 48 hours after undergoing a successful Roux-en-Y gastric bypass. A barium study reveals an anastomotic leak at the gastrojejunostomy anastomosis site. Which of the following is likely present in this patient?

A. Dilated loops of bowel
B. Unilateral pleural effusion
C. Decreased perfusion in the mesenteric arteries
D. Abnormality on EKG

276. A patient is started on 3 mg daily of oral semaglutide. The patient returns for follow-up lab work; the hemoglobin A1c is the same as it was before beginning semaglutide, three months prior. What is the reason for this lack of improvement?

    A. The starting dose has no glucose control
    B. This medication is only used for weight-loss
    C. This patient is a non-responder to therapy
    D. The hemoglobin A1c was checked too soon

277. A 16-year-old male is seen in the hospital on post-operative day one from a sleeve gastrectomy. In addition to abdominal pain, he complains of abdominal bloating, weakness, and dizziness while standing. Orthostatic vital signs are positive. What is the most appropriate test to order at this time?

    A. D-dimer
    B. Hemoglobin
    C. Chest x-ray
    D. Basic metabolic panel

278. A 39-year-old female with a past medical history of obesity class II and familial hypercholesteremia presents for follow-up after increasing her semaglutide level to the maximum dose for weight loss. Which of the following side effects is she most likely to be experiencing?

    A. Constipation
    B. Cold intolerance
    C. Palpitations
    D. Hirsutism

279. Which of the following conditions is setmelanotide approved for?

    A. Albright hereditary osteodystrophy
    B. Angelman syndrome
    C. Congenital leptin deficiency
    D. Bardet-Biedl

280. A patient presents to discuss different dietary options. She is particularly interested in initiating a low-fat diet. Which of the following is the most important piece of information to provide?

A. Target a reduction in your polyunsaturated intake
B. Replace saturated fats with refined carbohydrates
C. A lower-fat diet increases total cholesterol but decreases LDL
D. Replace saturated fats with whole grains

281. A study is being performed correlating increased percent body fat in those with metabolic syndrome. A direct correlation is found among different ethnic groups. Comparatively, which population would have higher rates of metabolic syndrome?

A. African American men
B. Hispanic women
C. Caucasian women
D. Asian men

282. A 46-year-old with recurrent migraines is presenting to discuss treatment options. She has tried topiramate but did not tolerate the side effects at the dose required to prevent migraines effectively. She is adamant about not wanting to start a medication that causes weight gain. Which of the following would be contraindicated, given her wishes?

A. Erenumab
B. Botox injections
C. Valproic acid
D. Zonisamide

283. An abdominal waist circumference is being performed on a patient prior to a referral to a renal transplant program. How should this measurement be completed to yield the most accurate results?

A. The measuring tape should be taut and compress the skin
B. The measurement should be done at the level of the iliac crest
C. The measurement should be done right after normal inspiration
D. The measuring tape should be at the level of the umbilicus

284. A 39-year-old female presents as an acute visit to the bariatric surgeon's office. The patient had undergone a Roux-en-Y gastric bypass three weeks prior. For the past five days she has had epigastric abdominal pain and progressively worsening nausea and vomiting. Vital signs are unremarkable. A barium study and upper endoscopy were unremarkable. Laboratory work, including a complete blood count, was normal. What is the most likely etiology of her symptoms?

A. Anastomotic leak
B. Mesenteric thrombosis
C. Marginal ulcer
D. Intraabdominal abscess

285. In studying neurohormonal interactions, it is found that a specific second-order neuron within the paraventricular nucleus leads to decreased weight. This describes which of the following?

A. Proopiomelanocortin
B. Agouti-related peptide
C. Melanin-concentrating hormone
D. Alpha melanocyte-stimulating hormone

286. A patient is discussing his difficulty breaking an eating pattern that he has had for the past 5 years. The patient is a realtor and takes himself out to a steakhouse every time he sells a house. He has become more successful than when he first started and now is finding himself going out to eat multiple times per week. Which area of the brain is responsible for this eating pattern?

A. Limbic system
B. Hippocampus
C. Homeostatic center
D. Amygdala

287. When was lorcaserin (Belviq®) taken off the market and why?

A. 1990 due to serotonin syndrome
B. 1997 due to heart valve problems
C. 2020 due to increased cancer risks
D. 2022 due to increased risk of pancreatitis

288. An 8-year-old female is diagnosed with Bardet-Biedl syndrome and a discussion of treatment options ensues. If started on setmelanotide, which of the following is a potential side effect?

    A. Nephrolithiasis
    B. Tachycardia
    C. Gastroparesis
    D. Skin hyperpigmentation

289. Which of the following is most important prior to metabolic and bariatric surgery?

    A. Delay surgery until a HbA1c of <8% is maintained
    B. Adherence to a 6-month dietary plan
    C. Screen all surgical patients with a TSH
    D. Avoid hormonal therapy 3 weeks prior to surgery

290. A 14-year-old female is on the maximum dose of phentermine/topiramate ER for weight loss and has lost 5% of her total body weight. Unfortunately, her father recently lost his job, including insurance coverage, and this medication is no longer affordable. Which of the following is a potential complication the daughter may experience if abruptly discontinued?

    A. Depression
    B. Seizure
    C. Rapid heartbeat
    D. Paresthesia

291. A 67-year-old male is following up from a motor vehicle accident in which the patient was ejected from the car, requiring emergent neurosurgery for a frontal epidural hematoma six months prior. The patient complains of erectile dysfunction, weight gain, frequent headaches, and cold intolerance since the accident. Which is the most likely cause of this patient's excess weight?

    A. Post-traumatic stress disorder
    B. Hypothalamic obesity
    C. Central hypothyroidism
    D. Hypogonadotropic hypogonadism

292. A patient is undergoing a bioelectrical impedance analysis at her initial obesity medicine consultation. Which of the following in her history would reduce the accuracy of this test?

A. Eating food before the test
B. Taking hydrochlorothiazide daily
C. History of alcohol use disorder
D. Exercising the day prior

293. A 32-year-old female with a history of diabetes type II and obesity class I presents to the emergency department after experiencing a seizure. Her glucose level on arrival was 18 mg/dL (reference range: 70–110 mg/dL), which responded well to dextrose. She is post-ictal and cannot provide a medical history, however, her husband states she was recently prescribed tirzepatide. Which other medication was she most likely taking?

A. Glipizide
B. Sitagliptan
C. Semaglutide
D. Empagliflozin

294. An 11-year-old female presents to the office for a well-child check. Her BMI is in the 90th percentile. She has no risk factors and otherwise feels well. What is the weight loss goal of this patient?

A. 1 lb weight loss per week
B. 2 lb weight loss per week
C. 1 lb weight loss per month
D. Weight maintenance

295. A 24-year-old female presents to the clinic. She states she goes to bed at midnight and sleeps until 9 am. She is a computer programmer and sits at her computer for 8 hours, only taking a short break for lunch. She drinks 3 cups of coffee daily. Her only medical condition is hypothyroidism, treated with levothyroxine. Which of the following places her at an increased risk of cardiovascular disease?

A. Career
B. Sleep pattern
C. Hypothyroid disease
D. Coffee consumption

296. A 19-year-old male has undergone a Roux-en-Y gastric bypass seven months ago and returns for follow-up after having abdominal pain, nausea, and right shoulder pain after meals. He occasionally eats fast food for convenience but has reduced portions. He has lost 65 lbs (29.5 kg) since surgery. Which of the following is most likely the cause of his symptoms?

A. Anatomic ulceration
B. Biliary colic
C. Internal hernia
D. Small intestine bowel overgrowth

297. A 9-year-old male presents for a well-child check. His BMI is in the 92nd percentile. What would be the best way to discuss this with the patient?

A. Can you tell me what types of foods you like to eat?
B. Would you mind if I ask you some questions about your body weight?
C. I am concerned about your BMI. Is this something you have thought about?
D. How do you feel about discussing a dietary and exercise plan today?

298. A 19-year-old female presents for a follow-up regarding polycystic ovarian syndrome (PCOS). A medical student asks the provider about the reason for decreased sex hormone binding globulin (SHBG) in this condition. What is the most accurate response?

A. Hyperinsulinism decreases hepatic SHBG production
B. Free androgens negatively feedback on estrogen production
C. Theca cells produce estrogen, which lowers SHBG levels
D. PCOS has high levels of SHBG, not low levels

299. Of the following medications used for weight loss, which is most likely to have an adverse effect on blood pressure?

A. Naltrexone
B. Phentermine
C. Bupropion
D. Topiramate

300. A 21-year-old female is trying to quit smoking before she becomes pregnant. She has unreliable transportation and the nearest location to purchase cigarettes is two miles away. During your discussions, it is recommended to no longer purchase cartons of cigarettes but rather buy only one pack at a time. What behavioral therapy component is this?

A. Goal setting
B. Stimulus control
C. Reward
D. Self-monitoring

Answer Explanations

Test Content Outline

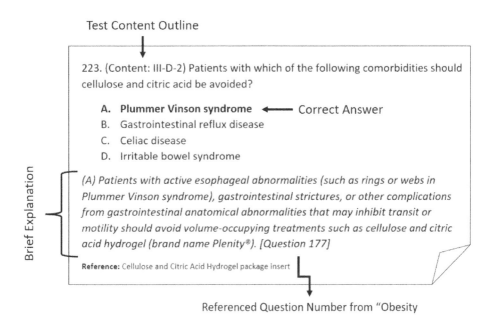

223. (Content: III-D-2) Patients with which of the following comorbidities should cellulose and citric acid be avoided?

A. **Plummer Vinson syndrome** ⟵ Correct Answer
B. Gastrointestinal reflux disease
C. Celiac disease
D. Irritable bowel syndrome

(A) Patients with active esophageal abnormalities (such as rings or webs in Plummer Vinson syndrome), gastrointestinal strictures, or other complications from gastrointestinal anatomical abnormalities that may inhibit transit or motility should avoid volume-occupying treatments such as cellulose and citric acid hydrogel (brand name Plenity®). [Question 177]

Reference: Cellulose and Citric Acid Hydrogel package insert

Brief Explanation

Referenced Question Number from "Obesity Medicine Board Review Questions, 2023"

95

1. (Content: III-D-2) A patient with end-stage renal disease on hemodialysis is presenting to a bariatric clinic for weight loss to become eligible for a renal transplant. Medications are discussed in detail. Which is the most appropriate treatment to start at this time?

    A. Semaglutide
    B. Naltrexone/buproprion ER
    C. Phentermine/topiramate ER
    D. Cellulose and Citric Acid Hydrogel

(A) In those with end-stage renal disease, orlistat, semaglutide, and liraglutide can be used in selected patients. Cellulose and citric acid hydrogel is not systemically absorbed and thus approved at any GFR. Semaglutide has increased weight loss potential compared to cellulose and citric acid hydrogel. [Question 108]

Reference: AACE/ACE Guidelines: AMERICAN ASSOCIATION OF CLINICAL ENDOCRINOLOGISTS AND AMERICAN COLLEGE OF ENDOCRINOLOGY COMPREHENSIVE CLINICAL PRACTICE GUIDELINES FOR MEDICAL CARE OF PATIENTS WITH OBESITY (2016): Recommendation 83-85

2. (Content: III-F-5c) A patient presents to a dermatologist with follicular hyperkeratosis. She had a malabsorptive procedure six years ago and admits to poor nutritional intake. Which vitamin or mineral, if replaced, would most likely improve her symptoms?

    A. Vitamin A
    B. Vitamin E
    C. Zinc
    D. Selenium

(A) Vitamin A deficiency can lead to night blindness and follicular hyperkeratosis. [Question 139]

Reference: AACE/TOS/ASMBS/OMA/ASA 2019 Guidelines: CLINICAL PRACTICE GUIDELINES FOR THE PERIOPERATIVE NUTRITION, METABOLIC, AND NONSURGICAL SUPPORT OF PATIENTS UNDERGOING BARIATRIC PROCEDURES – 2019 UPDATE. Recommendation 57, 62, 63-65

3. (Content: I-D-2) A patient takes supplemental folate. Where is the location of absorption for this vitamin?

A. Duodenum
B. Jejunum
C. Ileum
D. Colon

(B) The jejunum is a primary source of folate, carbohydrates, amino acids, and potassium absorption. The proximal portion of the jejunum can absorb iron as well. [Question 33]

Reference: Up to Date: "Bariatric surgery: Postoperative nutritional management"

4. (Content: III-F-5 and III-D-3) A 44-year-old female undergoes a workup for delayed post-prandial hypoglycemia two years after undergoing a gastric bypass. She is ultimately diagnosed with post-gastric bypass hypoglycemia and undergoes dietary changes without an improvement in symptoms. Which class of medications is indicated?

A. Complex disaccharides
B. Beta-blockers
C. Sulfonylureas
D. Biguanides

(A) Initial treatment of post-gastric bypass hypoglycemia should focus on dietary modifications with a low carbohydrate, mixed diet. Pharmacotherapy can be considered if these conservative measures are ineffective, including acarbose (complex disaccharide), octreotide (somatostatin analog), calcium channel blockers, or diazoxide. [Questions 149 and 167]

Reference: Rariy CM, Rometo D, Korytkowski M. Post-Gastric Bypass Hypoglycemia. Curr Diab Rep. 2016 Feb;16(2):19. doi: 10.1007/s11892-015-0711-5. PMID: 26868861.

5. (Content: III-F-5b) A 49-year-old male underwent a Roux-en-Y gastric bypass two years prior. He has taken vitamins intermittently. His vitamin D level is low and appropriate supplementation is initiated. What should be his maintenance dose?

A. 1000 IU daily
B. 2000 IU daily
C. 50000 IU weekly
D. A dose to maintain levels > 30 ng/mL

(D) Although 2000-3000 IU of vitamin D is recommended after metabolic surgery, the dose should be titrated to maintain a vitamin D level > 30ng/mL. This will vary with each patient. [Question 159]

Reference: AACE/TOS/ASMBS/OMA/ASA 2019 Guidelines: CLINICAL PRACTICE GUIDELINES FOR THE PERIOPERATIVE NUTRITION, METABOLIC, AND NONSURGICAL SUPPORT OF PATIENTS UNDERGOING BARIATRIC PROCEDURES – 2019 UPDATE. Recommendation 39.

6. (Content: II-B-4) A 44-year-old female consumes 40% of her calories in the evening when she returns home from work. In the morning, she denies hunger and often skips breakfast. What other finding is most likely present?

A. Sense of lack of control over eating
B. Increased dietary carbohydrate: protein ratio
C. Parasomnia
D. Purging behaviors after eating episodes

(B) Night eating syndrome is classically characterized by the triad of morning anorexia, evening hyperphagia, and insomnia. It is associated with nocturnal food consumption, increased carbohydrate-to-protein ratio (7:1), and consumption of 25-50% of daily calories after the evening meal. [Question 85]

Reference: Allison KC, Tarves EP. Treatment of night eating syndrome. Psychiatr Clin North Am. 2011;34(4):785–796. doi:10.1016/j.psc.2011.08.002

7. (Content: III-F-4) A 29-year-old female has completed her bariatric evaluation and is planning to undergo a sleeve gastrectomy within the next six months. She is currently on oral contraceptives. When should her contraceptive pills be stopped before surgery?

A. Right now
B. **One month prior**
C. One week prior
D. Continue these perioperatively

(B) Estrogen birth control should be stopped 1 cycle before surgery to prevent deep venous thrombosis (pre-menopausal), and hormone replacement therapy should be stopped 3 weeks prior in post-menopausal patients. [Question 192]

Reference: AACE/TOS/ASMBS/OMA/ASA 2019 Guidelines: CLINICAL PRACTICE GUIDELINES FOR THE PERIOPERATIVE NUTRITION, METABOLIC, AND NONSURGICAL SUPPORT OF PATIENTS UNDERGOING BARIATRIC PROCEDURES – 2019 UPDATE. Recommendation 14, 17, 18, 23

8. (Content: II-A-1 and II-B-5) A 21-year-old female presents to the clinic for evaluation of an IUD placement. Poor dentition and calluses over her knuckles are noted on the physical exam. She appears withdrawn and does not want to discuss other preventative measures. Which of the following statements is most accurate regarding her underlying condition?

A. Prevalence is equal among males and females
B. There are no FDA-approved pharmacologic treatments
C. BMIs are often in the underweight range
D. **Patients have a higher prevalence of prior sexual abuse**

(D) Bulimia affects up to 10% of women over their lifetime, with 16-22 year olds being the most common age group affected. The vast majority are females (90%), often with a concurrent mood disorder or history of abuse, especially sexual abuse (25%). [Questions 77 and 78]

Reference: Up To Date: "Eating disorders: Overview of prevention and treatment"
Reference: DSM-5: Diagnostic and Statistical Manual of Mental Disorders, Fifth Edition

9. (Content: I-A-3) A 7-year-old boy with a history of leptin deficiency is treated with appropriate medication. Two months later, he returns to the clinic, and his weight is reduced by 20 lbs (9.1 kg). Which of the following central hormones was likely inhibited after the initiation of treatment?

    A. Proopiomelanocortin
    B. Alpha melanocyte-stimulating hormone
    C. Cocaine and amphetamine-regulated transcript
    D. Orexin A and B

(D) Treatment with exogenous leptin in patients with leptin deficiency causes drastic weight loss by activating the anorexigenic pathway and inhibiting the orexigenic pathway (particularly neuropeptide Y, agouti-related peptide, and orexin A and B). [Question 19]

Reference: Varela L, Horvath TL. Leptin and insulin pathways in POMC and AgRP neurons that modulate energy balance and glucose homeostasis. EMBO Rep. 2012;13(12):1079-1086. doi:10.1038/embor.2012.174
Reference: Up to Date: "Physiology of leptin"

10. (Content: IV-A-1) A physician works alongside a physician assistant (PA) in a busy primary care clinic. The PA notices that most of the patients the physician assigns to him for the day have a BMI > 40 kg/m², whereas the patients the physician sees are generally of a normal BMI. The physician seems unaware of this pattern. This is an example of which of the following principles?

    A. Prejudice
    B. Stigma
    C. Implicit bias
    D. Malpractice

(C) Implicit bias occurs when the person is unaware of their deep-rooted views, often affecting how they act or treat an individual. This physician appears to have a preference for treating those with a normal BMI rather than those with obesity. [Question 217]

Reference: Puhl RM, Heuer CA. Obesity stigma: important considerations for public health. Am J Public Health. 2010;100(6):1019-1028. doi:10.2105/AJPH.2009.159491

11. (Content: III-D-2) A 39-year-old patient presents to a family practice clinic with complaints of brittle hair and cold intolerance. She has a history of hypothyroidism but has been stable on her dose for three years. She does admit to going to a weight loss clinic and being prescribed an anti-obesity medication. Which of the following weight-loss medications explains her presenting symptoms?

   A. **Orlistat**
   B. Semaglutide
   C. Phentermine
   D. Buproprion ER

(A) Orlistat can impair the absorption of levothyroxine. These medications should be spaced out four hours apart. [Question 132]

Reference: Orlistat package insert

12. (Content: II-D-2) For a small cost, a kiosk at the mall measures body fat percentages via bioelectrical impedance analysis (BIA) or calipers. Which of the following patients should BIA be recommended for testing over calipers?

   A. **BMI > 45 kg/m^2**
   B. Presence of a cardiac pacemaker
   C. Patient with decompensated cirrhosis
   D. Patient with poor skin turgor

(A) Bioelectrical impedance analysis is relatively accurate, inexpensive, and commonly used. It is hydration-dependent (best for euvolemic patients) and should be avoided if the patient has an electrical cardiac device. Calipers are user-dependent (variability) and not accurate at high BMI levels. [Question 50]

Reference: Obesity Medicine Association: Obesity Algorithm (2021)

13. (Content: I-B-4) A 43-year-old female with class III obesity is referred to the lymphedema clinic. Her lower extremity physical examination findings most likely include which of the following?

    A. Cuff sign
    B. "Round pea" sensation
    C. **Stemmer's sign**
    D. Lipodystrophy

(C) Stemmer's sign can help differentiate between lymphedema and lipedema. A negative Stemmer's sign occurs when you can grasp thin skin by pinching the upper surface of the second toe (lipedema). A positive test is when you can only grasp a lump of tissue (lymphedema), not the thin skin. [Question 11]

Reference: Okhovat JP, Alavi A. Lipedema: A Review of the Literature. Int J Low Extrem Wounds. 2015;14(3):262-267. doi:10.1177/153473461455428A

14. (Content: I-B-6 and 8) A 54-year-old male has made many dietary changes in the past year. He denies having time for physical activity but states his job "keeps him active." He has lost nearly 35 lbs (15.9 kg) during this time. He says he recently felt more hungry and has started to graze in the evenings. This has caused nearly 10 lbs (4.5 kg) in weight regain during the past two months. What mechanism is likely the culprit for his recent weight changes?

    A. **Neurohurmonal influences**
    B. Adaptive thermogenesis
    C. Set-point fallacy
    D. Increased muscle efficiency

(A) After patients lose weight, leptin, cholecystokinin, and peptide YY decrease, thus removing inhibitory actions on ghrelin; therefore, appetite often increases. [Questions 40 and 45]

Reference: Obesity medicine association: Obesity Algorithm (2021)
Reference: Erin E. Kershaw, Jeffrey S. Flier, Adipose Tissue as an Endocrine Organ, The Journal of Clinical Endocrinology & Metabolism, Volume 89, Issue 6, 1 June 2004, Pages 2548–2556, https://doi.org/10.1210/jc.2004-0395

15. (Content: III-F-1) A patient asks about realistic expectations that could be obtained after a Roux-en-Y gastric bypass. The average percentage of total body weight loss in 1 year is approximately

    A. 20-25%
    B. 25-30%
    C. 30-35%
    D. 35-40%

(C) Total body weight loss for different bariatric surgical options include gastric band 20-25%, sleeve gastrectomy 25-30%, Roux-en-Y gastric bypass 30-35%, and duodenal switch 35-45%. [Question 164]

Reference: AACE/TOS/ASMBS/OMA/ASA 2019 Guidelines: CLINICAL PRACTICE GUIDELINES FOR THE PERIOPERATIVE NUTRITION, METABOLIC, AND NONSURGICAL SUPPORT OF PATIENTS UNDERGOING BARIATRIC PROCEDURES – 2019 UPDATE. Table 6a.

16. (Content: II-C-4) Which is the most appropriate way to obtain the most accurate blood pressure?

    A. Rest the arm comfortably by the side
    B. Ensure clothes underneath the cuff is not bunched up
    C. The cuff bladder should encircle 80% of the arm circumference
    D. Distract the patient by talking with them

(C) Accurate blood pressure monitoring is important in diagnosing hypertension. Proper technique includes ensuring the patient is seated comfortably, with the back supported and the legs uncrossed. In addition, the blood pressure cuff should be on bare skin, the patient's arm should be supported at the heart level, the cuff bladder should encircle 80% of the arm circumference, and there should be no talking while obtaining the measurement. [Question 66]

References: New AHA Recommendations for Blood Pressure Measurement; Am Fam Physician. 2005 Oct 1;72(7):1391-1398.
Reference: 2017 ACC/AHA/AAPA/ABC/ACPM/AGS/APhA/ASH/ASPC/NMA/PCNA Guideline for the Prevention, Detection, Evaluation, and Management of High Blood Pressure in Adults

17. (Content: I-A-3) A 4-year-old with excess weight is being evaluated. When reviewing the chart, it is noted that the patient was treated in the NICU after birth due to profound hypotension. This patient most likely carries a defect in which gene?

A. **Proopiomelanocortin**
B. Leptin receptor
C. Melanocortin receptor
D. Orexin gene

(A) Proopiomelanocortin gene mutations lead to an adrenal crisis in neonatal life due to ACTH deficiency, which is produced from POMC (hypothalamus) as well as alpha-melanocyte-stimulating hormone, which is involved in reducing food intake. [Question 2]

Reference: Up To Date: "Genetic contribution and pathophysiology of obesity"

18. (Content: III-D-9) Which of the following comorbidities should be treated with bupropion in a patient with excess weight?

A. General anxiety disorder
B. Alcohol use disorder
C. Tics
D. **Seasonal affective disorder**

(D) A patient's comorbidities should be considered when prescribing anti-obesity medications, as there may be dual indications. For example, bupropion is used for smoking cessation, major depression disorder, and seasonal affective disorder. [Question 213]

Reference: Up to Date: "Obesity in adults: Drug therapy"

19. (Content: II-B-5) A 19-year-old female has recently been diagnosed with body dysmorphic syndrome. She states it is related to the excess adipose tissue on her stomach, of which she was bullied in high school by students telling her she looked pregnant. Since then, she has joined a gym and works on abdominal crunches for 2 hours daily. Which of the following is consistent with her condition?

    A. **Constantly asking friends for their opinions on her abdomen**
    B. Avoidance of mirrors or viewing herself in pictures
    C. Preoccupation with other peoples' similarly enlarged abdomens
    D. Diagnosis of concurrent bulimia nervosa

(A) The diagnostic criteria for body dysmorphic disorder include a preoccupation with ≥ 1 flaw in physical appearance that is not observable or appears slight to others that causes distress/impairment in areas of functioning. Repetitive behaviors seen in this condition include mirror checking, excessive grooming, skin picking, seeking reassurance, and comparing their appearance with others. [Question 90]

Reference: DSM-5: Diagnostic and Statistical Manual of Mental Disorders, Fifth Edition

20. (Content: I-B-1) Which of the following is the most accurate mechanism of ghrelin?

    A. **Stimulates NPY/AgRP receptors**
    B. Suppresses gut motility to promote absorption
    C. Increases energy expenditure
    D. Stimulates insulin secretion

(A) Ghrelin increases hunger by stimulating the orexigenic pathway through NPY/AgRP receptors in the central nervous system and, to some extent, through the vagal nerve. [Question 28]

Reference: Miller GD. Appetite Regulation: Hormones, Peptides, and Neurotransmitters and Their Role in Obesity. Am J Lifestyle Med. 2017;13(6):586-601. Published 2017 Jun 23. doi:10.1177/1559827617716376

21. (Content: III-F-3) Which of the following findings is more characteristic of an anastomotic ulcer when compared to a stricture following a Roux-en-Y gastric bypass?

A. Diagnosis involves an upper barium evaluation
B. Treatment includes endoscopic procedures
C. Pain is more localized within the abdomen
D. Symptoms can progress to dysphagia

(C) An anastomotic ulcer presents with more localized pain and commonly occurs due to risk factors, including anti-inflammatories, smoking, steroid use, and H. Pylori. It is diagnosed with an EGD and treated with lifestyle changes (i.e., smoking cessation, etc.) and proton pump inhibitors. [Question 154]

Reference: Obesity medicine association: Obesity Algorithm (2021)

22. (Content: III-D-2 and 9) A patient who admits to being addicted to soda is recently started on a medication to help with soda aversion, as it alters carbonic anhydrase on the tongue. What is the mechanism of this medication?

A. Stimulation of the hypothalamus to release norepinephrine
B. Enhancement of GABA activity and sodium channels
C. Agonist of glucagon-like 1 peptide receptor
D. Neuronal reuptake inhibition of norepinephrine and dopamine

(B) Topiramate alters the taste of carbonated beverages due to carbonic anhydrase inhibition and may be used for soda aversion. Although the exact mechanism of topiramate for weight loss is not well understood, it is theorized to enhance GABA activity and Na⁺ channels, leading to appetite suppression and satiety enhancement. [Questions 105 and 213]

Reference: Phentermine/topiramate ER package insert
Reference: Topiramate package insert.
Reference: Up to Date: "Obesity in adults: Drug therapy"

23. (Content: II-B-4) A 34-year-old businessman presents for therapy following a psychiatric evaluation. He is pursuing the gastric sleeve to cut down on the large meals he eats in a short duration of time. He admits he becomes embarrassed when he finishes his meal before his colleagues at meetings. What condition does he likely meet the criteria for?

  A. Night eating syndrome
  B. Major depressive disorder
  C. Binge eating disorder
  D. Body dysmorphic syndrome

(C) Binge eating disorder is a compulsive eating disorder characterized by marked distress about eating large amounts of food in a discrete amount of time with a sense of lack of control over eating during these episodes. It is associated with eating more rapidly than usual, until uncomfortably full, when not physically hungry, and hiding eating behaviors due to embarrassment. They often feel disgusted, depressed, or guilty after episodes. [Question 46]

Reference: DSM-5: Diagnostic and Statistical Manual of Mental Disorders, Fifth Edition

24. (Content: III-A-1) OARS is an acronym used in the setting of motivational interviewing. What does the 'R' stand for in this acronym?

  A. Reiterate
  B. Rapport
  C. Reflection
  D. Readiness

*(C) OARS is an acronym for **O**pen-ended questions, **A**ffirmation, **R**eflection, and **S**ummarize. [Question 186]*

Reference: Obesity medicine association: Obesity Algorithm (2021)

25. (Content: II-E, II-F, and II-A-3) A patient classified as stage 3 on the Edmonton Obesity Staging System (EOSS) would likely have which of the following comorbidities?

   A. **Suicidal ideation related to weight**
   B. Hypertension
   C. End-stage renal disease from diabetes
   D. Pre-diabetes

(A) The Edmonton Obesity Staging System (EOSS) is used to categorize patients based on the severity of obesity-related comorbidities, psychologic symptoms, and functional limitations rather than focusing strictly on anthropometric measurements such as waist circumference and body mass index. Stage 3 is characterized by significant obesity-related comorbidities with significant limitations, end-organ damage, or impairment, such as myocardial infarction, suicidal ideation, reduced mobility, stroke, and diabetic complications. [Questions 68 and 84]

Reference: Using the Edmonton obesity staging system to predict mortality in a population-representative cohort of people with overweight and obesity. Raj S. Padwal, Nicholas M. Pajewski, David B. Allison and Arya M. Sharma. CMAJ October 04, 2011 183 (14) E1059-E1066; DOI: https://doi.org/10.1503/cmaj.110387
Reference: "Assessment of obesity beyond body mass index to determine benefit of treatment." E. T. Aasheim, S. J. B. Aylwin, S. T. Radhakrishnan, A. S. Sood, A. Jovanovic, T. Olbers, C. W. le Roux, First published: 05 July 2011 https://doi.org/10.1111/j.1758-8111.2011.00017.x

26. (Content: I-A-3) Which of the following is considered an autosomal recessive cause of early-onset childhood obesity?

   A. **Congenital leptin deficiency**
   B. Prader-Willi syndrome
   C. MC4R deficiency
   D. Beckwith-Wiedemann syndrome

(A) Bardet-Biedl syndrome, POMC deficiency, congenital leptin deficiency, and Cohen syndrome (8q22 mutation) are autosomal recessive causes of early-onset childhood obesity. [Question 38]

Reference: Up to Date: "Beckwith-Wiedemann Syndrome"
Reference: Obesity medicine association: Pediatric Obesity Algorithm (2020-2022)

27. (Content: I-C-1 and 2) The rate of those diagnosed with excess weight continues to increase in the American population. Which of the following statements is most accurate?

A. 70% of adults have a BMI $\geq$30 kg/m^2
B. 1 in 3 children have obesity
C. 4 out of 10 adults meet the criteria for obesity
D. Rates of class III obesity has decreased in children

(C) Obesity is the most common chronic disease in the U.S. with 42.5% of adults having obesity (BMI $\geq$ 30 kg/m^2) and nearly 73.6% being overweight or meeting criteria for obesity (BMI $\geq$ 25 kg/m^2). [Questions 10 and 16]

Reference: https://www.cdc.gov/nccdphp/dnpao/data-trends-maps/index.html
Reference: CDC: https://www.cdc.gov/obesity/data/childhood.html#Prevalence

28. (Content: I-D-1) A 22-year-old presents to the emergency department by the police due to concerns about an inability to care for herself. She weighs 79 lbs (35.8 kg) and is concerned that she weighs too much. She has only consumed one large vegan salad daily for the past six months. What is likely seen on examination?

A. Abdominal fluid wave
B. Folate deficiency
C. Vitamin C deficiency
D. Tachycardia

(A) Kwashiorkor, a severe <u>protein</u> malnourishment, causes anasarca with ascites. Patients are typically apathetic and may have stripes in the hair (flag sign) on physical examination. Weight is variable, as protein deficiency may be countered by fluid weight from anasarca. [Question 25]

Reference: Up to Date: "Malnutrition in children in resource-limited countries: Clinical assessment"

29. (Content: III-F-5b) A 64-year-old female underwent a laparoscopic adjustable gastric banding (LABG) 6 years prior and has had minimal follow-up. She now states that she is having considerable abdominal pain. She says she can eat whatever she wants without feeling full. On physical examination, the port site appears red, with purulence noted. Which of the following is the most likely diagnosis?

A. Anastomotic leak
B. **Band erosion**
C. Gastric pouch dilation
D. Band slippage

(B) A potential complication after LABG is an erosion, which may be asymptomatic and present as a loss of food restriction or with findings of pain or infection at the port site. [Question 195]

Reference: AACE/TOS/ASMBS/OMA/ASA 2019 Guidelines: CLINICAL PRACTICE GUIDELINES FOR THE PERIOPERATIVE NUTRITION, METABOLIC, AND NONSURGICAL SUPPORT OF PATIENTS UNDERGOING BARIATRIC PROCEDURES – 2019 UPDATE. Recommendation 78
Reference: Obesity medicine association: Obesity Algorithm (2021)

30. (Content: II-C-3) A 33-year-old female presents with facial plethora and new-onset diabetes. On physical examination, she has a dorsal fat pad. Which of the following is the most critical next step in determining the etiology of her presentation?

A. **Medication review**
B. Cancer screening
C. Adrenal imaging
D. Dexamethasone suppression testing

(A) Cushing syndrome is characterized by facial plethora, moon/round face, dorsal fat pad (buffalo hump), hypertension, truncal obesity (thin extremities), proximal muscle weakness, osteoporosis, glucose intolerance, acne, and ecchymosis. The most common cause of hypercortisolism is iatrogenic. [Question 55]

Reference: Up to Date: "Establishing the diagnosis of Cushing's syndrome"

31. (Content: III-F-3) A patient successfully underwent a Roux-en-Y gastric bypass but now has recurrent episodes of tachycardia, facial flushing, abdominal cramping, and diarrhea after eating larger meals. What is the best next step for this patient?

    A. Screen for undiagnosed carcinoid syndrome
    B. Avoidance of foods with high concentrations of fats
    C. Increase protein intake
    D. Perform a breath hydrogen test

(C) Dumping syndrome presents with abdominal pain, cramping, tachycardia, diarrhea, and facial flushing due to high carbohydrate loads that rapidly empty into the small bowel. Dietary modifications are the preferred initial treatment with reduced carbohydrates (especially simple sugars), high-protein intake, increased dietary fiber, and changing to smaller, more frequent meals. [Question 119]

Reference: Up to Date: "Laparoscopic Roux-en-Y gastric bypass"

32. (Content: III-G-7) A patient was recently diagnosed with binge eating disorder. The only FDA medication specifically approved for this condition is also approved for which of the following?

    A. Depression
    B. Chronic migraines
    C. Untreated obstructive sleep apnea
    D. Attention deficit disorder

(D) Lisdexamfetamine dimesylate is the only FDA-approved for BED and attention-deficit/hyperactivity disorder. [Question 115]

Reference: Up To Date "Binge eating disorder in adults: Overview of treatment"

33. (Content: II-D-1) What is the respiratory quotient of proteins?

A. 0.7
B. 0.8
C. 1
D. 1.2

(B) The respiratory quotient allows you to determine which macronutrients are being consumed for energy in a steady state. The respiratory quotient for carbohydrates is 1, protein is 0.8, and fats are 0.7. [Question 56]

Reference: Patel H, Kerndt CC, Bhardwaj A. Physiology, Respiratory Quotient. 2020 Sep 16. In: StatPearls. Treasure Island (FL): StatPearls Publishing; 2021 Jan–. PMID: 30285389.

34. (Content: III-H-1 and III-D-6) A patient with previously poor nutrition decides to increase fiber intake with both dietary supplements and an increased intake of vegetables and fruits. What effect is this likely to have?

A. Resolution or improvement of acne
B. Improvements in cholesterol
C. Increased desire for energy-dense foods
D. Decreased risk of atrial fibrillation

(B) Fiber has many benefits, including improved blood glucose levels, reduced total cholesterol, reduced LDL cholesterol, improved satiety, and decreased constipation (via stool-bulking). In addition, studies have shown a reduced desire for energy-dense food intake and an increased desire for nutrient-rich foods with increased fiber intake. [Question 103]

Reference: Expert Panel on Integrated Guidelines for Cardiovascular Health and Risk Reduction in Children and Adolescents Full Report. Published Oct 2012.

35. (Content: III-G-4) An example of primary prevention for the development of obesity would include which of the following options?

A. Providing behavioral therapy interventions in an obesity clinic
B. Supplying free dietary plans for those with sleep apnea
C. Presenting pharmacotherapy options at a bariatric seminar
D. Sponsoring a day camp for youth focused on physical activity

(D) Primary prevention refers to preventing disease through education, screenings, and enacting preventative lifestyle modifications. [Question 98]

Reference: AACE/ACE Guidelines: AMERICAN ASSOCIATION OF CLINICAL ENDOCRINOLOGISTS AND AMERICAN COLLEGE OF ENDOCRINOLOGY COMPREHENSIVE CLINICAL PRACTICE GUIDELINES FOR MEDICAL CARE OF PATIENTS WITH OBESITY (2016): Recommendation 2

36. (Content: II-C-3 and I-B-4) A 13-year-old male with class II obesity presents with a limp with walking. He states he has been trying to exercise more but is limited by his pain. He is diagnosed with slipped capital femoral epiphysis. What would likely be seen on x-ray imaging?

A. Salter-Harris fracture
B. Bowing of the tibia
C. Avascular necrosis of the femoral head
D. Increased ossification of the tibial tuberosity

(A) Slipped capital femoral epiphysis (SCFE) results from the instability of the growth plate of the proximal femur, resulting in a Salter-Harris fracture. This is most commonly from fat mass disease (i.e., mechanical overload), although it can also be from a growth spurt. It requires urgent surgical evaluation. [Question 74]

Reference: Up to Date: Evaluation and Management of Slipped Capital Femoral Epiphysis (SCFE)

37. (Content: III-G-1) A 73-year-old female wants to start an exercise and dietary plan after a "wake-up call" with a recent myocardial infarction. Which of the following would be most appropriate to recommend as part of her regimen to prevent sarcopenia?

  A. **One hundred grams of protein intake daily**
  B. Total calorie intake of ≤ 1200 kcal/day
  C. Daily aerobic stationary bicycle riding
  D. Calcium and vitamin D supplementation

(A) Sarcopenia, or muscle loss, is a predisposing condition to eventual frailty, characterized by weight loss (often lean body mass), weakness, and reduced physical activity levels. Treatment recommendations include adequate protein intake (1-1.5 g/kg/day), resistance exercise training, and adequate vitamin and mineral supplementation. [Question 128]

Reference: Morley JE. Treatment of sarcopenia: the road to the future. J Cachexia Sarcopenia Muscle. 2018;9(7):1196-1199. doi:10.1002/jcsm.12386

38. (Content: I-B-2) Theoretically, a person who has a normal body mass index, when compared to a person with an elevated BMI, has increased levels of which of the following in the gastrointestinal tract?

  A. Prebiotic secretion
  B. Energy harvesting
  C. **Bacteroides**
  D. Firmicutes

(C) The two most common gut bacteria are Firmicutes and Bacteroides, comprising 92% of gut flora. In general, those who are leaner have higher levels of Bacteroides and decreased levels of Firmicutes than those affected by obesity. [Question 7]

Reference: Clarke SF, Murphy EF, Nilaweera K, et al. The gut microbiota and its relationship to diet and obesity: new insights. Gut Microbes. 2012;3(3):186-202. doi:10.4161/gmic.20168

39. (Content: II-B-5) A 19-year-old female is brought into the emergency department after passing out during a competitive dance competition. On arrival, she is alert and oriented, has poor skin turgor, and has temporal wasting. Her heart rate is 52/min. Based on the most likely diagnosis, which other findings would be appreciated?

A. Lack of concern about her low weight
B. Body mass index of 19 kg/m^2
C. Peaked T waves on an electrocardiogram
D. Pitting edema and anasarca

(A) Anorexia nervosa diagnostic criteria include restriction of energy intake relative to requirements leading to decreased weight, intense fear of gaining weight or becoming overweight or persistent behavior that interferes with weight gain, and body image distortion with a lack of recognition of the seriousness of the decreased weight. [Question 61]

Reference: DSM-5: Diagnostic and Statistical Manual of Mental Disorders, Fifth Edition

40. (Content: II-B-4) A pediatrician diagnoses a male patient with a condition similar to binge eating disorder seen in adult patients. Which of the following characteristics is likely present in this patient?

A. Apathy regarding his eating patterns
B. Tanner Stage 2
C. Purging after large meals
D. Symptoms ongoing for two months

(B) Loss of control eating disorder is nearly identical to binge eating disorder but is only diagnosed in children < 12 years old. [Question 70]

Reference: Tanofsky-Kraff M, Marcus MD, Yanovski SZ, Yanovski JA. Loss of control eating disorder in children age 12 years and younger: proposed research criteria. Eat Behav. 2008;9(3):360–365. doi:10.1016/j.eatbeh.2008.03.002

41. (Content: II-D-1) A laboratory monitors caloric utilization by different organ systems. Of the following, which would have the highest caloric requirements in a resting individual?

 A.   Heart
 B.   Kidney
 C.   Fat
 D.   Brain

(D) Skeletal muscle and the liver comprise the most substantial portion of the components that make up resting metabolic rate (RMR), accounting for 20% of RMR each. The brain accounts for 15%, the heart and digestive system are 10% each, and the kidneys and fat are 5% each. [Question 86]

Reference: Reference: Obesity medicine association: Obesity Algorithm (2021)

42. (Content: III-A-1) A 28-year-old female presents to discuss her prior weight loss attempts. She states she drinks four sodas daily and eats out almost daily for convenience. She says she finds it impossible to imagine not having these eating patterns. Which of the following phrases would be most appropriate at his time?

 A.   Why do you think you cannot change?
 B.   It sounds like you need some family support
 C.   You seem motivated to make some changes
 D.   Why do you drink that much soda in a day?

*(A) OARS is an acronym commonly used as a motivational interviewing skill that leads to higher patient engagement and ownership, decreasing resistance/barriers and improving overall outcomes. The **R** in **OARS** stands for reflection, which includes careful listening, facilitating evocation, developing discrepancy, resolving ambivalence, offering collaboration, and supporting self-efficacy. [Question 110]*

Reference: Obesity Medicine Association: Obesity Algorithm (2021)

43. (Content: II-C-6) A 24-year-old previously healthy female begins exercising 2-3 hours per day to gain muscle mass. She eats 6-12 raw egg whites daily for increased protein. If she continues this regimen, which vitamin deficiency is she most prone to develop?

A. Thiamine
B. Riboflavin
C. Biotin
D. Folate

(C) Consumption of a large quantity of raw egg whites can bind to biotin, preventing its absorption, and leading to a deficiency. Biotin deficiency can lead to facial dermatitis and neurologic findings (depression, neuropathy, hallucinations). [Question 65]

Reference: Up to Date: "Overview of water-soluble vitamins"

44. (Content: I-B-7) During an esophagogastroduodenoscopy, a biopsy of the duodenum is completed. Specialized testing reveals an anorexic hormone secreted from the K-cells. What hormone is being secreted?

A. Glucagon-like peptide 1
B. Cholecystokinin
C. Peptide YY
D. Glucose-dependent insulinotropic peptide

(D) Glucose-dependent insulinotropic peptide, also known as gastric inhibitory peptide, (GIP) is secreted by the duodenum and jejunum (K-cells) and has an insulin incretin effect and slows gastric emptying. [Question 1]

Reference: Miller GD. Appetite Regulation: Hormones, Peptides, and Neurotransmitters and Their Role in Obesity. Am J Lifestyle Med. 2017;13(6):586-601. Published 2017 Jun 23. doi:10.1177/1559827617716376

45. (Content: III-F-3) A patient underwent a successful laparoscopic Roux-en-Y gastric bypass and is 8 hours post-operative. The nurse notices darker urine despite adequate intraoperative fluid administration. Which intraoperative risk factors likely contributed to this patient's condition?

A. **Length of surgery**
B. Biliary duct injury
C. Traumatic Foley insertion
D. Reaction to medications

(A) Rhabdomyolysis can occur in the setting of prolonged surgery, with severe obesity being a risk factor. Muscle breakdown can occur as the patient's body lies on the minimally padded operating room table. [Question 123]

Reference: Up to Date: "Clinical manifestations and diagnosis of rhabdomyolysis"

46. (Content: III-D-7) A pediatrician is interested in prescribing medications for weight loss. Based on her comfort level, she does not want to prescribe any medications off-label. Which of the following weight-loss medications would be an option for her?

A. Metformin in a 12-year-old
B. **Liraglutide in a teenager**
C. Phentermine for a 6-month duration in a 17-year-old
D. Naltrexone/bupropion ER in a 15-year-old

(B) Most obesity medications are approved for adults only. The exceptions are phentermine in those ≥ 16 years old (considered off-label if used for ≥3 months) and orlistat, phentermine/topiramate ER, and liraglutide (Saxenda®) in those ≥12 years old. In addition, Setmelanotide is approved in those as young as 6 years old for POMC, PCSK1, or LEPR mutations, and Bardet-Biedl syndrome. Semaglutide is likely to be approved for those ≥12 years old soon. [Question 146]

Reference: Up to Date: "Overweight and obesity in adults: Health consequences"

47. (Content: III-D-8) A psychiatrist is treating a patient with new-onset bipolar disorder. The patient has class II obesity and is concerned about medication-induced weight gain. Which of the following is the most weight-neutral mood stabilizer?

    A. Divalproex
    B. Lithium
    C. Gabapentin
    D. Lamotrigine

(D) Weight-positive mood stabilizers include divalproex, lithium, and carbamazepine. In contrast, weight-neutral/variable options include lamotrigine (possibly weight-negative) and oxcarbazepine. [Question 204]

Reference: Obesity medicine association: Obesity Algorithm (2021)

48. (Content: III-H-1) A 9-year-old male presents to a multidisciplinary weight loss center. Laboratory work will be obtained during this visit. When would it be most appropriate to obtain liver enzymes to screen for metabolic-associated fatty liver disease (MAFLD)?

    A. If the patient's weight is in the 90th percentile with a diagnosis of prediabetes
    B. On any patient with a BMI greater than the 85th percentile
    C. Regardless of BMI, if the parents have a history of MAFLD
    D. If the patient's weight is at the 94th percentile

(A) Liver enzymes should be obtained in pediatric patients when the BMI is in the 85th- 94th percentile with risk factors (prediabetes/diabetes, hyperlipidemia, sleep apnea, central adiposity, or family history of metabolic-associated fatty liver disease) or in anyone with a BMI ≥ 95th percentile. [Question 95]

Reference: Expert Committee Recommendations Regarding the Prevention, Assessment, and Treatment of Child and Adolescent Overweight and Obesity: Summary Report and APPENDIX. Sarah E. Barlow and the Expert Committee; Pediatrics December 2007, 120 (Supplement 4) S164-S192; DOI: https://doi.org/10.1542/peds.2007-2329C.

49. (Content: III-G-2) How would ursodeoxycholic acid be used in the management of patients with obesity?

A. To prevent the progression of fatty liver disease
B. Dissolve formed gallstones after bariatric surgery
C. To treat dumping syndrome post Roux-en-Y gastric bypass
D. Prevent cholecystectomy after gastric bypass surgery

(D) Cholelithiasis can occur from rapid weight loss after bariatric surgery and ursodeoxycholic acid may prevent this complication. It does not have evidence to support its use if stones are already formed preoperatively. [Question 180]

Reference: AACE/TOS/ASMBS/OMA/ASA 2019 Guidelines: CLINICAL PRACTICE GUIDELINES FOR THE PERIOPERATIVE NUTRITION, METABOLIC, AND NONSURGICAL SUPPORT OF PATIENTS UNDERGOING BARIATRIC PROCEDURES – 2019 UPDATE. Recommendation 72-75
Reference: Ursodeoxycholic acid for the prevention of symptomatic gallstone disease after bariatric surgery (UPGRADE): a multicentre, double-blind, randomised, placebo-controlled superiority trial. Lancet gastroenterol Hepatol. 2021 Dec;6(12):993-1001. doi: 10.1016/S2468-1253(21)00301-0. Epub 2021 Oct 27. PMID: 34715031.

50. (Content: II-C-7) Using growth charts based on the percentile of body mass index is best in which of the following cohorts?

A. Neonatal period
B. Once a child begins walking
C. Those over the age of 2
D. Tanner Stage 2 and above

(C) Weight assessment in those under 2 years old is done by evaluating weight for length using the World Health Organization charts, taking into account gender and age. In contrast, percentile of body mass index is not used until after two years of age. [Question 83]

Reference: https://www.cdc.gov/growthcharts/who_charts.htm

51. (Content: III-G-2) A 51-year-old female presents for her annual evaluation after undergoing a successful Roux-en-Y gastric bypass three years prior. She states that she has had frequent yeast infections within the skin folds of her abdomen despite trying to keep them clean and dry. Which of the following is the most appropriate solution to this problem?

A. Oral fluconazole
B. Topical nystatin cream
C. Referral to plastic surgery
D. Topical clindamycin

(C) Intertrigo and recurrent yeast infections after significant weight loss are not uncommon given the excess skin that may be present. An abdominoplasty can be done for both psychosocial and physical health reasons and is a long-term solution in those with recurrent infections. Although treating the infection with topical nystatin is appropriate, it is a short-term fix instead of a long-term solution. This patient should be referred to plastic surgery to discuss and determine if body contouring surgery would be appropriate. [Question 129]

Reference: Sadeghi P, Duarte-Bateman D, Ma W, Khalaf R, Fodor R, Pieretti G, Ciccarelli F, Harandi H, Cuomo R. Post-Bariatric Plastic Surgery: Abdominoplasty, the State of the Art in Body Contouring. J Clin Med. 2022 Jul 25;11(15):4315. doi: 10.3390/jcm11154315. PMID: 35893406; PMCID: PMC9330885.

52. (Content: III-D-3) A patient was recently started on topiramate for idiopathic intracranial hypertension and weight loss (off-label). Which of the following lab abnormalities is expected with topiramate use?

A. Elevated triglycerides
B. Non-anion gap metabolic acidosis
C. Lactic acidosis
D. Hyperkalemia

(B) Hyperchloremic metabolic acidosis (non-anion gap metabolic acidosis) is associated with topiramate use. This medication can be used for several reasons off-label, including idiopathic intracranial hypertension, migraine prevention, and binge-eating disorder. [Question 203]

Reference: Topiramate package insert

53. (Content: III-F-5b) The most common long-term complication of laparoscopic adjustable gastric banding is

    A. band slippage
    B. erosion
    C. port issues
    D. **required revision/removal**

(D) Long-term complications of laparoscopic adjustable gastric banding include band slippage (3-5%), gastric pouch dilation (3-5%), erosion (1%), port issues (2-5%), and need for removal or revision for various reasons (25%). [Question 195]

Reference: AACE/TOS/ASMBS/OMA/ASA 2019 Guidelines: CLINICAL PRACTICE GUIDELINES FOR THE PERIOPERATIVE NUTRITION, METABOLIC, AND NONSURGICAL SUPPORT OF PATIENTS UNDERGOING BARIATRIC PROCEDURES – 2019 UPDATE. Recommendation 78
Reference: Obesity medicine association: Obesity Algorithm (2021)

54. (Content: III-D-6) A 36-year-old male presents to the emergency department with jaundice and darkened urine. On laboratory analysis, he is found to be in acute hepatic failure. He states he started a supplement that was supposed to help with increasing energy expenditure. Which of the following is most likely contributing to his presentation?

    A. **Yerba Mate**
    B. Guar gum
    C. Chitosan
    D. Hydroxycitric acid

(A) Supplements marketed to increase energy expenditure include yerba mate, ephedra, guarana, Yohimbe, country mallow, and bitter orange. [Question 109]

Reference: Up to Date: "Overview of herbal medicine and dietary supplements"

55. (Content: I-D-2) A patient starts cellulose and citric acid hydrogel to assist with weight loss. The hydrated capsules will eventually break down in the gastrointestinal tract, with water reabsorption occurring at what location?

    A. Duodenum
    B. Jejunum
    C. Ileum
    D. Colon

(D) The colon is the location for vitamin K, biotin, B_1, B_3, water, sodium, and chloride. [Question 33]

Reference: Up to Date: "Bariatric surgery: Postoperative nutritional management"
Reference: Cellulose and Citric Acid Hydrogel package insert

56. (Content: III-F-3) A 44-year-old male underwent a sleeve gastrectomy complicated by prior surgical adhesions and scarring, requiring conversion to an open surgery. Given the additional time for stomach resection, the surgery time lengthened significantly. Which of the following is likely to be increased on post-operative day one?

    A. Bicarbonate level
    B. Creatine phosphokinase
    C. Sodium and chloride
    D. Total bilirubin

(B) Rhabdomyolysis can occur in the setting of prolonged surgery, with severe obesity being a risk factor. Muscle breakdown can occur as the patient's body lies on the minimally padded operating room table. Diagnosis is confirmed with serum creatine phosphokinase (CPK) levels. To affect kidney function, CPK levels typically are > 10,000 IU/L, with decreased urine output being one of the initial findings. [Question 123]

Reference: Up to Date: "Clinical manifestations and diagnosis of rhabdomyolysis"

57. (Content: III-H-1 and 3 and III-F-6) A pediatric clinic is starting a weight management program where they can provide support through dieticians and physical therapists to provide motivational interviewing and monthly follow-up visits. Which of the following accurately describes the highest-tiered intervention they can provide?

A. Prevention
B. Prevention plus
C. **Structured weight management**
D. Comprehensive multidisciplinary intervention

(C) Stage 2 of the 4-tiered approach for management of pediatric obesity includes structured weight management in a primary care office, with support available (dieticians, therapist, etc.). Monthly follow-up is recommended. [Questions 130 and 197]

Reference: Expert Committee Recommendations Regarding the Prevention, Assessment, and Treatment of Child and Adolescent Overweight and Obesity: Summary Report. Sarah E. Barlow. Pediatrics Dec 2007, 120 (Supplement 4) S164-S192; DOI: 10.1542/peds.2007-2329C

58. (Content: III-D-8) A patient is establishing care with a new primary care physician. It is noted that metformin is on his medication list without a diagnosis of diabetes. The patient states that his psychiatrist started a medication that may cause weight gain and simultaneously prescribed metformin to reduce that side effect. What other medicine was this patient likely prescribed?

A. **Olanzapine**
B. Nortriptyline
C. Bupropion
D. Desvenlafaxine

(A) Metformin is proven effective (off-label) for antipsychotic-related weight gain. This medication should be considered when antipsychotics are initiated to prevent weight gain, which is generally more effective than adding it after weight gain has already occurred. [Question 193]

Reference: Metformin package insert.
Reference: (Baptista 2007; Chen 2013; Das 2012; de Silva 2016; Jarskog 2013; Wang 2012; Zheng 2015)

59. (Content: III-A-2) After discussing weight loss goals and preferences, a patient is encouraged to develop a SMART goal. In this acronym, what does the 'M' stand for?

    A. Measurable
    B. Meaningful
    C. Motivation
    D. Manageable

*(A) A **SMART** goal is an acronym for setting a quality and challenging goal. It stands for **S**pecific, **M**easurable, **A**chievable, **R**elevant, and **T**imed. [Question 214]*

Reference: Bovend'Eerdt TJ, Botell RE, Wade DT. Writing SMART rehabilitation goals and achieving goal attainment scaling: a practical guide [published correction appears in Clin Rehabil. 2010 Apr;24(4):382]. Clin Rehabil. 2009;23(4):352-361. doi:10.1177/0269215508101741

60. (Content: III-B-1 and 4) A 47-year-old female with hyperlipidemia and prediabetes presents to her primary care physician because she is not tolerating statin therapy. She would prefer to pursue dietary modifications rather than medication for primary cardiovascular prevention. She is planning to start on a low-carbohydrate or keto diet. Three months from now, how will her laboratory work change?

    A. Decreased HDL
    B. Increase in TG
    C. Increase in LDL
    D. Unchanged total cholesterol

(C) In general, low carbohydrate diets have more significant improvements in HDL and TG. There may be an increase in LDL, which may be very significant in those with genetic hypercholesterolemia. A ketogenic diet is associated with moderately increased LDL and total cholesterol, as carbohydrates are often exchanged for foods higher in cholesterol and saturated fats. Low carbohydrate diets do cause improvements in insulin resistance, glucose levels, and HbA1c irrespective of weight loss. [Question 174]

Reference: Obesity medicine association: Obesity Algorithm (2021)

61. (Content: III-G-7) A patient is being treated with cognitive behavioral therapy for a condition in which she eats excessively in a short amount of time and then has immense guilt. She hides her behaviors from her friends. Which of the following therapies would most likely be beneficial to her?

A. **Topiramate**
B. Buspirone
C. Bariatric surgery
D. Semaglutide

(A) While the only FDA-approved pharmacotherapy for BED is lisdexamfetamine dimesylate (brand name Vyvanse®), many medications are commonly used off-label and have good efficacy, including topiramate, phentermine/topiramate ER, selective serotonin reuptake inhibitors, and bupropion. [Question 115]

Reference: Up To Date "Binge eating disorder in adults: Overview of treatment"

62. (Content: II-D-3-b) A 21-year-old female presents to her primary care for follow-up regarding prior insulin resistance. She was recently started on metformin and initiated lifestyle changes. She has lost 2% of her body weight but states her menstrual cycles are still irregular. Which of the following findings was most likely present on her initial evaluation?

A. Dorsal fat pad
B. Unilateral adnexal enlargement
C. Seborrheic keratosis
D. **Adrenergic alopecia**

(D) Diagnosis of polycystic ovarian syndrome based on the Rotterdam Consensus states patients must meet 2 of the 3 for diagnosis: hyperandrogenism (biochemical or clinical), menstrual irregularities (anovulation), and polycystic ovaries by ultrasound. [Question 79]

Reference: Up to Date: "Diagnosis of polycystic ovary syndrome in adults"

63. (Content: III-F-3) A patient who underwent a successful Roux-en-Y gastric bypass presents for a one-month post-operative follow-up appointment. Although the patient has experienced weight loss, she states she is now unable to tolerate solid food and has reverted to a liquid diet. She felt like food was getting stuck. Which of the following is the most appropriate treatment for her condition?

A. Antibiotics
B. **Endoscopic procedure**
C. Anti-inflammatories
D. Laparoscopic revision

(B) Patients presenting with dysphagia and solid food intolerance after a gastric bypass should be evaluated for a stricture or stenosis. Treatment includes endoscopic balloon dilation, as surgical intervention is rarely indicated. [Question 154]

Reference: Obesity medicine association: Obesity Algorithm (2021)

64. (Content: II-C-1 and 5) Patients with which of the following conditions should consistently utilize special growth charts and BMI curves?

A. Down syndrome
B. Addison's disease
C. **Achondroplasia**
D. Congenital hypothyroidism

(C) Certain populations have unique pediatric BMI curves, including patients with achondroplasia. Although patients with Down syndrome have an increased risk of obesity and use different charts for weight and height, the BMI guidelines from the CDC recommend using charts for normally developing children to provide early detection of excess weight and incorporate early intervention. [Question 92]

Reference: Up to Date: Achondroplasia
Reference: Obesity medicine association: Pediatric Obesity Algorithm (2020-2022)

65. (Content: I-D-1) Which of the following is an essential amino acid?

A. Arginine
B. Methionine
C. Proline
D. Tyrosine

(B) Essential amino acids must be consumed, as the human body cannot make them. They include histidine, isoleucine, leucine, lysine, methionine, phenylalanine, threonine, tryptophan, and valine. [Question 25]

Reference: Up to Date: "Malnutrition in children in resource-limited countries: Clinical assessment"

66. (Content: IV-A-1) A nurse tells a physician that she received a call regarding one of his patients that was not tolerating one of her new blood pressure medications. The patient's BMI is 46 kg/m². The physician states, "She probably just doesn't want to take medicines; she never does anything I tell her." This attitude is an example of which of the following?

A. Stigma
B. Burnout
C. Implicit bias
D. Prejudice

(A) Stigma occurs when someone sees another person as having lower social value based on a physical or character trait. Importantly, stigma often occurs amongst physicians. Physicians self-report that they often view their patients with obesity as non-adherent, dishonest, lazy, unsuccessful, and lacking self-control. [Question 217]

Reference: Puhl RM, Heuer CA. Obesity stigma: important considerations for public health. Am J Public Health. 2010;100(6):1019-1028. doi:10.2105/AJPH.2009.159491

67. (Content: III-G-2) A 39-year-old male presents six months after a sleeve gastrectomy with complaints of debilitating gastroesophageal reflux in the evenings. He has tried dietary changes, sleeping in a recliner, and increasing omeprazole to twice daily without relief. A urease breath test and barium study is unremarkable. Which of the following would be appropriate at this time?

A. Add famotidine to his medicine regimen
B. Evaluate for a hiatal hernia with endoscopy
C. Initiate metoclopramide before meals
D. **Conversion to a Roux-en-Y gastric bypass**

(D) After sleeve gastrectomy, conversion to Roux-en-Y should be considered if patients develop severe GERD, which is recalcitrant to medical therapy. [Question 180]

Reference: AACE/TOS/ASMBS/OMA/ASA 2019 Guidelines: CLINICAL PRACTICE GUIDELINES FOR THE PERIOPERATIVE NUTRITION, METABOLIC, AND NONSURGICAL SUPPORT OF PATIENTS UNDERGOING BARIATRIC PROCEDURES – 2019 UPDATE. Recommendation 72-75

68. (Content: II-D-3a) A 44-year-old female with class III obesity presents to her primary care physician to review recent test results for daytime fatigue. She has hypertension controlled with chlorthalidone. She underwent a home polysomnography which showed no desaturations and minimal apneic events. Her blood work revealed significant respiratory acidosis. Her echocardiogram revealed minimally elevated right ventricular pressures without other abnormalities. Which of the following is the best next step in management?

A. **Trial a non-invasive positive airway pressure machine**
B. Repeat the polysomnography at a sleep facility
C. Order pulmonary function testing
D. Evaluate with a right heart catheterization

(A) Obesity hypoventilation syndrome (OHS) requires the following for diagnosis: Body mass index > 30 kg/m^2, PaCO$_2$ > 45 mmHg, and exclusion of other causes. First-line treatment is non-invasive positive airway pressure, whereas definitive treatment focuses on weight loss. [Question 94]

Reference: Up to Date: "Treatment and prognosis of the obesity hypoventilation syndrome"

69. (Content: I-B-4) A 19-year-old female presents to her primary care physician with the chief complaint of "being funny-shaped." In particular, she complains of needing to shop for larger pant sizes, but her shoe size is relatively small. What additional finding would be most likely?

A. Abdominal striae and easy bruising
B. History of lymph node dissection
C. Similar exam findings in her sister
D. Telangiectasias and caput medussa

(C) Lipedema is an abnormal subcutaneous fat deposition predominantly affecting the lower extremities. It commonly occurs in women, with onset between 15-30 years of age. It frequently is seen in other family members. [Question 11]

Reference: Okhovat JP, Alavi A. Lipedema: A Review of the Literature. Int J Low Extrem Wounds. 2015;14(3):262-267. doi:10.1177/153473461455428A

70. (Content: II-C-6) A patient presents with decreased sensation to monofilament testing and reduced vibratory sensations in the lower extremity bilaterally. These findings may be seen in which of the following water-soluble vitamin deficiencies?

A. B_2
B. B_3
C. B_6
D. B_9

(C) Pyridoxine deficiency (B_6) can cause symptoms that include peripheral neuropathy and microcytic anemia. [Question 65]

Reference: Up to Date: "Overview of water-soluble vitamins"

71. (Content: I-B-7) A company produces a synthetic high-potency hormone that suppresses glucagon production and increases satiety. What of the following hormones does this describe?

   A. Cholecystokinin
   B. Peptide YY
   C. Oxyntomodulin
   D. Glucagon-like peptide 1

(D) Glucagon-like peptide 1 (GLP-1) is secreted by the distal small bowel and colon (L-cells) and has an incretin effect in response to carbohydrate ingestion. This includes glucose-dependent insulin secretion, hepatic gluconeogenesis reduction via glucagon suppression, and delays in gastric emptying, leading to increased satiety and reduced appetite. [Question 1]

Reference: Miller GD. Appetite Regulation: Hormones, Peptides, and Neurotransmitters and Their Role in Obesity. Am J Lifestyle Med. 2017;13(6):586-601. Published 2017 Jun 23. doi:10.1177/1559827617716376

72. (Content: II-C-7) A 12-year-old female presents for a well-child visit. Which is the most accurate way of classifying her weight category?

   A. Weight-for-length
   B. Absolute BMI
   C. Percentile range of BMI
   D. Percentage of body fat

(C) In children ages 2-20, weight status is based on a <u>percentile</u> range of BMI, considering gender and age. [Question 59]

Reference: Obesity medicine association: Pediatric Obesity Algorithm (2020-2022)

73. (Content: II-B-4) A 19-year-old male with obesity presents for dietary counseling. He admits to working longer hours during the day and frequently snacks on potato chips, peanut butter sandwiches, and soda. When he gets home, he eats a significant amount of calories throughout the evening and occasionally wakes up in the night for a quick snack. Which of the following recommendations would have the most significant impact on his eating habits?

A. **Eat breakfast every morning**
B. Increase unsaturated fat intake to slow gastric emptying
C. Begin pharmacotherapy with phentermine
D. Change to wholegrain bread

(A) Night eating syndrome is classically characterized by the triad of morning anorexia, evening hyperphagia, and insomnia. Treatment is focused on encouraging regular meal consumption earlier in the daytime, with increased protein intake being very effective. [Question 85]

Reference: Allison KC, Tarves EP. Treatment of night eating syndrome. Psychiatr Clin North Am. 2011;34(4):785–796. doi:10.1016/j.psc.2011.08.002

74. (Content: II-D-1) In the setting of low-energy sustainable exercise (such as a slow jog in a marathon), if a steady state is maintained, the respiratory quotient will predominantly indicate burning which of the following elements?

A. Carbohydrates
B. Proteins
C. **Fats**
D. Fruits

(C) The respiratory quotient allows you to determine which macronutrients are consumed for energy in a steady state. If low-energy but sustainable exercise is being performed (jogging in a marathon), the RQ will be closer to 0.7, as stored fats are primarily used for energy. In addition, inactivity tends to be closer to 0.7. If high-intensity, high-energy exercise is being performed (sprinting), carbohydrates are mainly used for energy, and the RQ is near 1. [Question 56]

Reference: Patel H, Kerndt CC, Bhardwaj A. Physiology, Respiratory Quotient. 2020 Sep 16. In: StatPearls. Treasure Island (FL): StatPearls Publishing; 2021 Jan–. PMID: 30285389.

75. (Content: II-B-3) A couple decides to pursue a diet that avoids poultry and red meat. However, they plan to continue to eat salmon and almond milk. Which of the following diets does this describe?

A. Lacto-ova
B. Pescatarian
C. Vegan
D. Vegetarian

(B) Variants of the vegetarian-based diets include lacto-ova (consume dairy and eggs), pescatarian (eat fish, but no red meat or poultry), vegans (consume absolutely no animal products), and vegetarians (may eat animal products such as milk and eggs, but no meat). [Question 51]

Reference: Up to date: "Vitamin supplementation in disease prevention"

76. (Content: II-E, II-F, and II-A-3) What is the benefit of utilizing the Edmonton Obesity Staging System (EOSS) over anthropometric measurements such as waist circumference and body mass index (BMI)?

A. It is used to screen candidates for obstructive sleep apnea
B. Life insurance companies use it to determine surgery eligibility
C. It helps determine the long-term impact of obesity on a patient
D. It justifies bariatric surgery in those who do not meet BMI criteria

(C) The Edmonton Obesity Staging System provides better insight into the patient's long-term impact of obesity and may help determine the level of appropriate treatment (along with established metrics). It is used to categorize patients based on the severity of obesity-related comorbidities, psychologic symptoms, and functional limitations rather than focusing strictly on anthropometric measurements. [Questions 68 and 84]

Reference: Using the Edmonton obesity staging system to predict mortality in a population-representative cohort of people with overweight and obesity. Raj S. Padwal, Nicholas M. Pajewski, David B. Allison and Arya M. Sharma. CMAJ October 04, 2011 183 (14) E1059-E1066; DOI: https://doi.org/10.1503/cmaj.110387
Reference: "Assessment of obesity beyond body mass index to determine benefit of treatment." E. T. Aasheim, S. J. B. Aylwin, S. T. Radhakrishnan, A. S. Sood, A. Jovanovic, T. Olbers, C. W. le Roux, First published: 05 July 2011 https://doi.org/10.1111/j.1758-8111.2011.00017.x

77. (Content: II-B-5) A 16-year-old male is brought into the clinic for concerns of an eating disorder. Which of the following would best differentiate the eating disorder of bulimia from anorexia?

A. Fear of gaining weight
B. Compensatory behaviors
C. **Body mass index**
D. Self-image distortion

(C) The severity of anorexia nervosa is based on body mass index (BMI), with mild disease consisting of a BMI between BMI ≥ 17-18.5 kg/m². Patients with bulimia will often have a normal or increased BMI. [Question 61]

Reference: DSM-5: Diagnostic and Statistical Manual of Mental Disorders, Fifth Edition

78. (Content: I-A-4) A 51-year-old male presents with peripheral vision loss, headaches, and decreased sexual desire. Subsequent imaging shows a cystic structure in the pituitary stalk. Which of the following best describes this finding?

A. Prolactinoma
B. Pituitary macroadenoma
C. **Craniopharyngioma**
D. Optic glioma

(C) A craniopharyngioma is a rare, slow-growing cystic (sometimes solid) lesion that often arises from the remnants of Rathke's pouch. It can compress and damage pituitary and hypothalamic structures leading to hypogonadism, hypothyroidism, diabetes insipidus, and deficiencies of growth hormone and adrenocorticotropic hormone. Headaches and visual abnormalities are common. If suspected, an MRI of the brain should be obtained. Craniopharyngiomas are a cause of hypothalamic obesity. [Question 42]

Reference: Up To Date: "Craniopharyngioma" and "Obesity in adults: Etiologies and risk factors"

79. (Content: III-F-5a) A 29-year-old female is presenting for a one-week follow-up after undergoing a successful Roux-en-Y gastric bypass. Although she has discontinued her sliding scale insulin due to a hypoglycemic episode, she has had persistent post-prandial hyperglycemia of 180-200 mg/dL. Her medications for diabetes currently include metformin ER and maximally tolerated semaglutide. Which of the following would be the best pharmacologic management of her diabetes?

A. Resume a reduced insulin sliding scale
B. Stop metformin due to the risk of lactic acidosis
C. Change the metformin formulation
D. Initiate and up-titrate empagliflozin

(C) Metformin can be continued after gastric bypass, although metformin should be changed to immediate-release (IR) to increase absorption and bioavailability. After gastric bypass or sleeve gastrectomy, IR formulations are preferred, as the transit time within the stomach and proximal small intestines is reduced (sleeve gastrectomy) or this area is bypassed (RYGB). In addition, the risk of lactic acidosis from metformin is reduced after RYGB in the absence of renal dysfunction. [Question 160]

Reference: AACE/TOS/ASMBS/OMA/ASA 2019 Guidelines: CLINICAL PRACTICE GUIDELINES FOR THE PERIOPERATIVE NUTRITION, METABOLIC, AND NONSURGICAL SUPPORT OF PATIENTS UNDERGOING BARIATRIC PROCEDURES – 2019 UPDATE. Recommendation 42

80. (Content: III-D-8) Which antipsychotic medication would be most appropriate for a patient with excess weight?

A. Olanzapine
B. Ariprazole
C. Clozapine
D. Risperidone

(B) Most antipsychotic medications cause weight gain. The most weight-positive antipsychotic medications include olanzapine, lithium, quetiapine, clozapine, and risperidone. In contrast, aripiprazole, ziprasidone, and haloperidol tend to have less weight-gaining potential. [Question 204]

Reference: Obesity medicine association: Obesity Algorithm (2021)

81. (Content: I-A-3) A pharmacy receives a shipment of metreleptin. Which patient diagnosis is an indication for this therapy?

    A. Proopiomelanocortin gene mutations
    B. Congenital leptin deficiency
    C. PCSK1 genetic defect
    D. Melanocortin 4 receptor deficiency

(B) Setmelanotide is approved for Bardet-Biedl syndrome, as well as POMC and LEPR deficiency; leptin replacement therapy (metreleptin) is approved for congenital leptin deficiency with lipodystrophy. [Question 2]

Reference: Up To Date: "Genetic contribution and pathophysiology of obesity"

82. (Content: I-E-1) A patient begins a new exercise program utilizing boxing for cardiac aerobic therapy. The type of muscle fibers used in this program have which of the following properties?

    A. Has significantly higher levels of mitochondria
    B. Tends to be fatigue-resistant
    C. Is similar to the muscles used in triathlons
    D. Uses anaerobic glycolysis for metabolism

(D) Fast twitch (type II) muscle fibers are utilized in acceleration and speed, such as sprinting or boxing. These muscles primarily use anaerobic glycolysis for metabolism and are susceptible to fatigue. [Question 41]

Reference: Ørtenblad N, Nielsen J, Boushel R, Söderlund K, Saltin B, Holmberg HC. The Muscle Fiber Profiles, Mitochondrial Content, and Enzyme Activities of the Exceptionally Well-Trained Arm and Leg Muscles of Elite Cross-Country Skiers. Front Physiol. 2018;9:1031. Published 2018 Aug 2. doi:10.3389/fphys.2018.01031

83. (Content: III-F-1 and 2) An aspiration device is being offered at a bariatric surgery clinic. A patient with the following conditions would be a poor candidate to receive this therapy?

    A. Body mass index of 51 kg/m^2
    B. Significant mental disability
    C. A history of multiple C-sections
    D. Paraplegia of lower extremities

(B) The AspireAssist® is an FDA-approved, long-term weight loss device for adults ≥22 years old, with a BMI of 35-55 kg/m^2. Importantly, ensuring the patient is logistically able to perform the aspiration (schedules, mental capacity, time commitment, etc.) is vital for success. Other contraindications include a history of refractory stomach ulcers, esophageal strictures, severe gastroparesis, pregnancy (or breastfeeding), eating disorders, and physical/mental disability or psychologic illness that may interfere with adherence. [Questions 102 and 150]

Reference: Reference: AspireAssist® Clinician guide

84. (Content: I-B-1 and 7) An endogenous rectal hormone is synthetically produced and injected into mice. The mice have transient gastroparesis and increase the length of time between feedings. What hormone is being described?

    A. Glucagon-like peptide 1
    B. Oxyntomodulin
    C. Peptide YY
    D. Leptin

(C) Peptide YY is an endogenous hormone produced and secreted from the distal small bowel, colon, and rectum, acting as a natural potent appetite suppressant. In addition, it delays gastric and intestinal motility. [Questions 1 and 20]

Reference: Daily, intermittent intravenous infusion of peptide YY(3-36) reduces daily food intake and adiposity in rats. Prasanth K. Chelikani, Alvin C. Haver, Joseph R. Reeve Jr., David A. Keire, and Roger D. Reidelberger 01 Feb 2006; https://doi.org/10.1152/ajpregu.00674.2005 **Reference:** Miller GD. Appetite Regulation: Hormones, Peptides, and Neurotransmitters and Their Role in Obesity. Am J Lifestyle Med. 2017;13(6):586-601. Published 2017 Jun 23. doi:10.1177/1559827617716376

85. (Content: II-A-4) A 52-year-old male has been waking up in the middle of the night to eat food while still asleep. This has occurred approximately three times weekly over the past three months. The patient is most likely to have which of the following findings?

A. Periodic limb movement disorder
B. Orthostatic hypotension
C. Use of fluoxetine
D. Family history of dementia

(A) Sleep-related eating disorder (SRED) is a sleep-walking variant affecting approximately 3% of the general population. The majority of patients with SRED (80%) have associated restless leg syndrome (RLS), periodic limb movement disorder (PLMD), obstructive sleep apnea (OSA), or somnambulism. [Question 87]

Reference: Up To Date: "Disorders of arousal from non-rapid eye movement sleep in adults"

86. (Content: III-F-5c) A zinc deficiency could cause which of the following symptoms?

A. Anemia
B. Night blindness
C. Seborrheic dermatitis
D. Anosmia

(D) Zinc deficiency can cause alopecia, anosmia, brittle nails, and chronic diarrhea. In males, it can also cause hypogonadism or erectile dysfunction. [Question 139]

Reference: AACE/TOS/ASMBS/OMA/ASA 2019 Guidelines: CLINICAL PRACTICE GUIDELINES FOR THE PERIOPERATIVE NUTRITION, METABOLIC, AND NONSURGICAL SUPPORT OF PATIENTS UNDERGOING BARIATRIC PROCEDURES – 2019 UPDATE. Recommendation 57, 62, 63-65

87. (Content: II-C-5) A 2-year-old male with gross motor deficits presents with his parents to a nutritionist after recently gaining weight. Genetic testing reveals a paternal chromosome 15q partial deletion. Which of the following would likely be seen upon examining his hands?

    A. Normal fingers
    B. Polydactyly
    C. Shortened 4th and 5th metacarpal bones
    D. Brachydactyly

(A) Prader-Willi syndrome occurs due to a paternal chromosome 15q partial deletion (i.e., under-expressed gene). Physical examination findings include characteristic thin upper lips and almond-shaped eyes. Obesogenic conditions that affect the hands include Albright Hereditary Osteodystrophy (shortened 4th and 5th metacarpal bones), and Bardet-Biedl syndrome (polydactyly). *[Question 48]*

Reference: Cassidy SB, Driscoll DJ. Prader-Willi syndrome. Eur J Hum Genet. 2009;17(1):3-13. doi:10.1038/ejhg.2008.165
Reference: Up to Date: "Clinical features, diagnosis, and treatment of Prader-Willi syndrome"

88. (Content: III-A-1) An obesity medicine specialist meets with a new patient interested in behavioral modification related to weight loss. The physician states, "I understand it can be difficult to lose weight. Tell me about your history with trying to lose weight?" Which key process of motivational interviewing is being displayed?

    A. Evoking
    B. Planning
    C. Engagement
    D. Focusing

(C) Engagement is the key process of motivational interviewing that establishes a therapeutic relationship by displaying empathy and acceptance in addition to utilizing o*pen-ended questions,* a*ffirmation,* r*eflection, and* s*ummarizing (OARS). [Question 186]*

Reference: Obesity medicine association: Obesity Algorithm (2021)

89. (Content: I-C-1) The two most commonly acquired information for obesity rates and statistics is based on surveys from the National Health and Nutrition Examination Survey (NHANES) and the Behavioral Risk Factor Surveillance System (BRFSS). Which of the following statements on obesity surveying is most accurate?

A. BRFSS surveys are based on a larger sample size
B. NHANES surveys are based on self-reported weight data
C. BRFSS has consistently been more accurate with weight
D. NHANES surveys tend to over-report rates of obesity

(A) The NHANES survey does in-person weighing (smaller cohort) and is considered more accurate than the BRFSS survey, which is self-reported over the phone, and the participants tend to under-report weight. [Questions 10 and 16]

Reference: https://www.cdc.gov/nccdphp/dnpao/data-trends-maps/index.html

90. (Content: II-D-3b) A 44-year-old female presents to the clinic after losing nearly 13 lbs (5.9 kg) within the last three months. Her weight has been stable over the past five years before this recent weight loss. When would her level of sex hormone binding globulin (SHBG) be highest?

A. Now
B. Three months ago
C. Three years ago
D. Five years ago

(A) SHBG is decreased in patients with obesity. However, with weight loss, these levels will increase. SHBG also increases proportionally with age. [Question 91]

Reference: Zhu JL, Chen Z, Feng WJ, Long SL, Mo ZC. Sex hormone-binding globulin and polycystic ovary syndrome. Clin Chim Acta. 2019 Dec;499:142-148. doi: 10.1016/j.cca.2019.09.010. Epub 2019 Sep 13. PMID: 31525346.
Reference: Cooper LA, Page ST, Amory JK, Anawalt BD, Matsumoto AM. The association of obesity with sex hormone-binding globulin is stronger than the association with ageing--implications for the interpretation of total testosterone measurements. Clin Endocrinol (Oxf). 2015 Dec;83(6):828-33. doi: 10.1111/cen.12768. Epub 2015 May 11. PMID: 25777143; PMCID: PMC4782930.

91. (Content: II-C-7) What is most accurate regarding the cohort data from the Centers for Disease Control and Prevention (CDC) growth charts?

A. Data is based predominantly on breastfed children
B. These charts best reflect those between 0-2 years of age
C. The CDC charts should not be utilized in other countries
D. Data is based predominantly on Caucasians

(D) The CDC growth charts are based on a cohort of primarily non-breastfed, Caucasian American children. The CDC chart cohort data was not available for the first three months of age, and the sample sizes were limited for sex and age for the first six months. Thus, it is recommended to use the WHO growth standards for infants 0-2 years of age and the CDC growth charts after that. [Question 83]

Reference: https://www.cdc.gov/growthcharts/who_charts.htm

92. (Content: III-D-2) A 34-year-old female is interested in starting phentermine/topiramate ER after not meeting weight loss goals with lifestyle modifications alone. What would be the best question to ask before initiating this medication?

A. Can you remember to take medications twice daily?
B. Have you had any previous seizures?
C. Are you on any chronic pain medications?
D. Are you sexually active?

(D) All FDA-approved weight loss medications are contraindicated during pregnancy. In particular, topiramate causes an increased risk of birth defects, including cleft lips and cleft palates. If this medication is prescribed to women of child-bearing age, sexual activity and birth control must be discussed. [Question 105]

Reference: Phentermine/topiramate ER package insert

93. (Content: III-F-4) A patient is brought to the operating room before undergoing a sleeve gastrectomy procedure. The anesthesiologist finds out that the patient had a meal replacement shake 3 hours before the surgery and threatens to cancel the surgery. Which of the following would be the best response?

    A. "I agree. This patient is at high risk for aspiration."
    B. "The shake will help with post-operative bowel function."
    C. "If the shake was clear, it should be okay to continue with surgery."
    D. "Let's delay surgery for a few more hours."

(B) Preoperative enhanced recovery after bariatric surgery (ERABS) clinical pathways should be implemented in all patients undergoing bariatric surgery to improve postoperative outcomes. This includes allowing the patient to have oral nutrition with carbohydrates up to 2 hours preoperatively to decrease insulin resistance, decrease protein catabolism, reduce hospital length of stay, and experience a faster return of bowel function. [Question 111]

Reference: AACE/TOS/ASMBS/OMA/ASA 2019 Guidelines: CLINICAL PRACTICE GUIDELINES FOR THE PERIOPERATIVE NUTRITION, METABOLIC, AND NONSURGICAL SUPPORT OF PATIENTS UNDERGOING BARIATRIC PROCEDURES – 2019 UPDATE. Recommendation 34, 35, 36, 40. Table 8.

94. (Content: III-D-2) A 24-year-old female presents to the clinic for follow-up after starting an FDA-approved anti-obesity medication that causes decreased fat absorption. What is a potential complication of this medication?

    A. Thiamine deficiency
    B. Congenital birth defects
    C. Nephrolithiasis
    D. Cholelithiasis

(C) Orlistat can cause oxalate nephropathy. Normally, calcium would bind to oxalate in the intestines, both being excreted in the stool. In the presence of orlistat, fat absorption is decreased, allowing fat to bind to calcium, leaving oxalate unopposed, and increasing absorption. These high levels of oxalate can precipitate in the kidney. [Question 132]

Reference: Orlistat package insert

95. (Content: III-H-1) An 11-year-old female presents to her pediatrician for a follow-up regarding weight management. The patient's weight is in the 95th percentile, and blood pressure was elevated on the prior visit. Her mother has end-stage cirrhosis secondary to metabolic-associated fatty liver disease (MAFLD). Given the above findings, what is the best initial screening test for this patient?

- A. AST: ALT ratio
- **B. ALT**
- C. AST
- D. MAFLD fibrosis score

(B) In children with obesity, nearly 1/3 will have fatty liver disease, with ALT being the best initial screening test. Metabolic-associated fatty liver disease (MAFLD) has replaced the nomencleature of non-alcohol fatty liver (NAFLD) disease to better describe the underlying physiology. [Question 95]

Reference: Expert Committee Recommendations Regarding the Prevention, Assessment, and Treatment of Child and Adolescent Overweight and Obesity: Summary Report and APPENDIX. Sarah E. Barlow and the Expert Committee; Pediatrics December 2007, 120 (Supplement 4) S164-S192; DOI: https://doi.org/10.1542/peds.2007-2329C.

96. (Content: II-C-4) A 14-year-old adolescent with an arm circumference of 32 cm presents for a blood pressure evaluation. His blood pressure was elevated during a prior examination, although ambulatory home measurements were within normal limits. Which of the following cuff sizes is most appropriate for this patient?

- A. Pediatric (18-22 cm)
- B. Small adult (22-26 cm)
- **C. Adult (27-34 cm)**
- D. Large adult (45-52 cm)

(C) An appropriately sized blood pressure cuff for the patient's arm size is required for accurate measurements. The term "large adult" for a blood pressure cuff is a misnomer, as it should be based on the arm circumference, not adult size. [Question 66]

References: New AHA Recommendations for Blood Pressure Measurement; Am Fam Physician. 2005 Oct 1;72(7):1391-1398.
Reference: 2017 ACC/AHA/AAPA/ABC/ACPM/AGS/APhA/ASH/ASPC/NMA/PCNA Guideline for the Prevention, Detection, Evaluation, and Management of High Blood Pressure in Adults

97. (Content: II-B-4) Which of the following is most similar to loss of control eating disorder?

- A. Bulimia Nervosa
- B. Night eating syndrome
- C. Leptin deficiency
- **D. Binge eating disorder**

(D) Loss of control eating disorder is nearly identical to binge eating disorder but is only diagnosed in children < 12 years old. [Question 70]

Reference: Tanofsky-Kraff M, Marcus MD, Yanovski SZ, Yanovski JA. Loss of control eating disorder in children age 12 years and younger: proposed research criteria. Eat Behav. 2008;9(3):360–365. doi:10.1016/j.eatbeh.2008.03.002

98. (Content: III-H-4) Education is being provided to new foster parents of a 5-year-old regarding maintaining a healthy weight. Which of the following recommendations is most appropriate?

- A. Limit sugar-sweetened beverages to no more than one per day
- B. Breakfast should be limited to oatmeal, fruits, or eggs
- **C. An hour of physical activity is recommended daily**
- D. Children with 7-8 hours of sleep perform optimally during school

(C) Healthy lifestyle habits for children include healthy eating and decreasing sedentary time. This includes limiting screen time to 2 hours daily, encouraging sleeping ≥ 9 hours nightly, eating ≥ 5 servings of fruits and vegetables daily, minimizing or eliminating (preferred) sugar-sweetened beverages, preparing meals at home when possible, eating at the table with family ≥ 5 times weekly, consuming a healthy breakfast every morning, and performing at least 60 minutes of physical activity daily. [Question 100]

Reference: Expert Committee Recommendations Regarding the Prevention, Assessment, and Treatment of Child and Adolescent Overweight and Obesity: Summary Report.. Sarah E. Barlow and the Expert Committee; Pediatrics December 2007, 120 (Supplement 4) S164-S192; DOI: https://doi.org/10.1542/peds.2007-2329C.

99. (Content: I-B-1) The orexigenic hormone produced in the stomach would be at its peak levels in which scenario?

A. With increased adipose tissue
B. After the consumption of carbohydrates
C. Status post sleeve gastrectomy
D. During a stressed state

(D) Ghrelin is the only gastrointestinal orexigenic hormone made in the gastric fundus and body, as well as the proximal small intestines. Levels are increased in the setting of an empty stomach, fasting state, after weight loss, with stress or sleep deprivation, and Prader-Willi syndrome. [Question 28]

Reference: Miller GD. Appetite Regulation: Hormones, Peptides, and Neurotransmitters and Their Role in Obesity. Am J Lifestyle Med. 2017;13(6):586-601. Published 2017 Jun 23. doi:10.1177/1559827617716376

100. (Content: III-G-7) A 33-year-old Caucasian male presents to his primary care physician after gaining 45 lbs (20.4 kg) over the past year since working from home. His blood pressure has been persistently elevated, and he is agreeable to starting an anti-hypertensive medication while working on lifestyle changes. Which class of antihypertensive should be recommended?

A. Calcium channel blocker
B. Thiazide diuretic
C. Beta-blocker
D. Angiotensin receptor blocker

(D) Renin-angiotensin-aldosterone system (RAAS) *activation seems to be a primary mediator in hypertension in patients with obesity (especially in children). This is because pro-inflammatory adipokines released by excessive amounts of adipose tissue activate the sympathetic nervous system, ultimately activating RAAS, leading to aldosterone-mediated sodium and water absorption within the kidney. Blockade of this pathway is preferred for anti-hypertensives in patients with obesity. [Question 168]*

Reference: AACE/ACE Guidelines: AMERICAN ASSOCIATION OF CLINICAL ENDOCRINOLOGISTS AND AMERICAN COLLEGE OF ENDOCRINOLOGY COMPREHENSIVE CLINICAL PRACTICE GUIDELINES FOR MEDICAL CARE OF PATIENTS WITH OBESITY (2016). Recommendation 91-94.

101. (Content: II-D-3a) An 18-year-old female presents to her primary care physician for persistent headaches and occasional double vision. She states these occurred toward the end of her first semester of college. Since graduating high school, she has gained approximately 25 lbs (11.3 kg). Her eye doctor noted abnormalities on fundoscopic examination, although her corrective lenses are adequate. Her STOP-BANG score is 2. Which of the following is the most appropriate treatment?

A. Counseling regarding alcohol use
B. Carbonic anhydrase inhibitors
C. CPAP machine at night
D. Latanoprost eye drops

(B) Treatment options for idiopathic intracranial hypertension should include weight loss of >5-10% (lifestyle modifications and/or medical or surgical options) with a low sodium diet. In addition, carbonic anhydrase inhibitors such as acetazolamide and topiramate (which also helps with weight loss) lower cerebral fluid pressure. Surgical interventions such as optic nerve sheath fenestration and shunting procedures should be pursued in the setting of deteriorating vision or intractable headaches. [Question 58]

Reference: Up to Date: "Idiopathic intracranial hypertension (pseudotumor cerebri): Clinical features and diagnosis & prognosis and treatment"

102. (Content: III-D-2) Cellulose and citric acid hydrogel (brand name Plenity®) is approved for what minimum body mass index with no obesity-related comorbidity?

A. 23 kg/m^2
B. 25 kg/m^2
C. 27 kg/m^2
D. 30 kg/m^2

(B) Cellulose and citric acid hydrogel (brand name Plenity®) is a volume-occupying treatment for those with a BMI between 25-40kg/m^2. [Question 179]

Reference: Cellulose and Citric Acid Hydrogel package insert

103. (Content: III-F-3) A 59-year-old male presents to the emergency department due to dehydration and lack of oral nutrition. He is eight months status-post Roux-en-Y gastric bypass. He has lost nearly 85 lbs (38.6 kg) post-operatively but has developed intermittent abdominal pain and post-prandial satiety over the past two months. Over the last two days, his abdominal pain significantly increased, and he could not tolerate any oral intake. A CT scan shows a mesenteric swirl sign. Which of the following is the most likely diagnosis?

    A. Large bowel obstruction
    B. Volvulus
    C. Small bowel ileus
    D. Internal hernia

(D) Intermittent abdominal pain and postprandial satiety are concerning for a mesenteric defect causing an internal hernia. These symptoms often occur before a small bowel obstruction. The most specific CT finding for an internal hernia is a "mesenteric swirl sign." [Question 166]

Reference: Internal Hernia after Laparoscopic Gastric Bypass: A Review of the Literature; April 26, 2007 by Louis O. Jeansonne IV, MD; Craig B. Morgenthal, MD; Brent C. White, MD; and Edward Lin, DO

104. (Content: III-A-1) A 37-year-old patient is considering quitting smoking within the next month. He wanted to discuss strategies that are used to help with the process. This patient is most likely in which of the following stages of change?

    A. Pre-contemplation
    B. Contemplation
    C. Preparation
    D. Action

(C) The stages of change include pre-contemplation, contemplation, preparation, action, and maintenance. Preparation refers to the willingness to change in the next 30 days (planning). [Question 116]

Reference: Obesity Medicine Association: Obesity Algorithm (2021)

105. (Content: III-F-2) A patient has been recommended to undergo tarsal tunnel surgery, but the podiatrist will not perform the surgery until the patient has lost 5% of his weight. The patient has not lost enough weight with extensive lifestyle changes alone and wishes to discuss weight loss options, including placing a gastric balloon. Which of the following recommendations is most appropriate?

A. **Plan for tarsal tunnel surgery six months after the balloon is placed**
B. The balloon is unlikely to reduce weight by 5%
C. A BMI of 34 kg/m^2 does not meet the criteria for a balloon
D. If used appropriately, balloons have a high risk of deflation and bowel obstruction

(A) Intragastric balloons are a short-term option (6 months maximum) in adults with a body mass index of 30-40 kg/m^2 and one or more obesity-related comorbidity in those who failed lifestyle modifications. They have proven short-term effectiveness, ranging from a 6.8%-10.2% decrease in body weight. [Question 176]

Reference: Up to Date: "Intragastric balloon therapy for weight loss"
Reference: Reshapelifesciences.com and Obera.com

106. (Content: III-F-3) A 34-year-old female underwent a bariatric surgery complicated by intrabdominal adhesions from prior C-sections and laparoscopic cholecystectomy. The patient is difficult to wean from the ventilator, with oxygen desaturations and increased respiratory rate when placed on spontaneous breathing. Which of the following is the most likely cause?

A. **Venous thromboembolism**
B. Obesity hypoventilation syndrome
C. Obstructive sleep apnea
D. Rhabdomyolysis

(A) Patients who are difficult to wean from the vent should make you consider pulmonary embolisms and anastomotic leaks. [Question 133]

Reference: AACE/TOS/ASMBS/OMA/ASA 2019 Guidelines: CLINICAL PRACTICE GUIDELINES FOR THE PERIOPERATIVE NUTRITION, METABOLIC, AND NONSURGICAL SUPPORT OF PATIENTS UNDERGOING BARIATRIC PROCEDURES – 2019 UPDATE. Recommendation 45, 46

107. (Content: III-A-1) During a weight management discussion, a physician documents a weight loss plan, including specific goals discussed during the visit. Which action does this describe based on the 5 A's of obesity management?

A. Assess
B. Advise
C. Agree
D. Assist

(C) 'Agree' is the component of the 5 A's of obesity management (ask, assess, advise, agree, arrange/assist) related to agreeing on realistic weight-loss goals and expectations and documenting specific details of the agreed-upon treatment plan. [Question 147]

Reference: Obesity medicine association: Obesity Algorithm (2021)

108. (Content: I-B-5) Indirect calorimetry would best help determine which of the following metabolic parameters?

A. Resting energy expenditure
B. Non-exercise activity thermogenesis
C. Thermic effect of meals
D. Energy expenditure from physical activity

(A) Indirect calorimetry can help determine the basal metabolic rate, as it is used as a proxy for resting energy expenditure. [Question 4]

Reference: Obesity medicine association: Obesity Algorithm (2021)

109. (Content: III-F-5c) A female presents to her primary care physician with numbness and weakness in the lower extremities. Physical examination reveals an abnormal gait with sensory ataxia. What nutritional deficiency does this describe?

A. Riboflavin
B. Copper
C. Niacin
D. Zinc

(B) A deficiency of copper can cause anemia, neutropenia, myeloneuropathy, and impaired wound healing. Myeloneuropathy can present with ataxia/spasticity, neuropathy, and weakness. [Question 139]

Reference: AACE/TOS/ASMBS/OMA/ASA 2019 Guidelines: CLINICAL PRACTICE GUIDELINES FOR THE PERIOPERATIVE NUTRITION, METABOLIC, AND NONSURGICAL SUPPORT OF PATIENTS UNDERGOING BARIATRIC PROCEDURES – 2019 UPDATE. Recommendation 57, 62, 63-65

110. (Content: III-A-1) A psychologist is using motivational interviewing skills in a multidisciplinary obesity medicine clinic. The patient has lost 10 lbs (4.5 kg) in the past four weeks but does admit to still eating fast food 1-2 times weekly. Which of the following statements or questions reflect the principle of supporting self-efficacy?

A. "What can you do to maintain this rate of weight loss in the future?"
B. "Your weight loss could be even more impressive if you avoided fast food."
C. "Your weight loss in the past four weeks shows your motivation."
D. "What skills do you think were most influential in your successful weight loss?"

(C) In motivational interviewing, the principle of supporting self-efficacy refers to affirming favorable results by focusing on the patient's successes, skills, and strengths. [Question 161]

Reference: Obesity medicine association: Obesity Algorithm (2021)

111. (Content: I-B-6) A biologist is studying relative hormone levels secreted by adipose tissue. It is determined that the most abundant hormone synthesized and released by adipose tissue

   A.   increases aromatase conversion of estrogen
   B.   enhances insulin sensitivity and skeletal glucose uptake
   C.   increases inflammation within the vascular endothelium
   D.   slows down gastrointestinal motility

(B) Adiponectin is exclusively produced by white adipose tissue and is the most abundantly produced and secreted hormone from adipose tissue. It enhances insulin sensitivity, fatty acid oxidation, and decreases gluconeogenesis within the liver; it also increases fatty acid oxidation and glucose uptake within skeletal muscles. Adiponectin also reduces inflammation, particularly within the endothelium of the vasculature. [Question 17]

Reference: Erin E. Kershaw, Jeffrey S. Flier, Adipose Tissue as an Endocrine Organ, The Journal of Clinical Endocrinology & Metabolism, Volume 89, Issue 6, 1 June 2004, Pages 2548–2556, https://doi.org/10.1210/jc.2004-0395

112. (Content: III-D-8) Which of the following is a contraindication for metformin use?

   A.   Prior Roux-en-Y gastric bypass
   B.   Concurrent diastolic heart failure
   C.   A patient over the age of 70 years old
   D.   A patient on peritoneal dialysis

(D) Contraindications to metformin include hypersensitivity to metformin, eGFR < 30 mL/min, or acute or chronic metabolic acidosis. [Question 193]

Reference: Metformin package insert.
Reference: (Baptista 2007; Chen 2013; Das 2012; de Silva 2016; Jarskog 2013; Wang 2012; Zheng 2015)

113. (Content: I-B-7) Which of the following hormones is a long-acting signaling hormone that increases in the setting of excess adiposity?

A. Orexin
B. Leptin
C. Adiponectin
D. Glucagon

(B) Leptin has a role in central signaling regarding energy sufficiency. As adipose tissue increases, leptin increases, thus signaling satiety and increasing energy expenditure. Its levels are proportionate to body fat mass. [Question 29]

Reference: Erin E. Kershaw, Jeffrey S. Flier, Adipose Tissue as an Endocrine Organ, The Journal of Clinical Endocrinology & Metabolism, Volume 89, Issue 6, 1 June 2004, Pages 2548–2556, https://doi.org/10.1210/jc.2004-0395

114. (Content: III-D-3) Naltrexone/bupropion ER should be avoided in patients with which of the following characteristics?

A. A history of opioid use disorder
B. A blood pressure of 160/90 mmHg
C. A history of calcium oxalate nephrolithiasis
D. A history of depression

(B) Contraindications to naltrexone/bupropion ER include hypersensitivity to bupropion or naltrexone, uncontrolled hypertension, seizure disorder, history of seizures, risk of seizures (bulimia, anorexia nervosa, alcohol or benzo withdrawal, etc.), chronic current opioid use, pregnancy, and concurrent use of MAO-I. [Question 181]

Reference: Naltrexone/bupropion ER package insert

115. (Content: II-B-4) An 11-year-old female with a diagnosis of obesity class I presents to her pediatrician at her mother's urging. For the past six months, she has been stashing a significant amount of food in her room and rapidly eating it. The rest of the day, she looks defeated and is very irritable. Which of the following is the most effective management for her likely condition?

A. Psychotherapy
B. Metformin
C. Topiramate
D. Group therapy

(A) Interpersonal psychotherapy is the first-line treatment for loss of control eating disorder. [Question 70]

Reference: Tanofsky-Kraff M, Marcus MD, Yanovski SZ, Yanovski JA. Loss of control eating disorder in children age 12 years and younger: proposed research criteria. Eat Behav. 2008;9(3):360–365. doi:10.1016/j.eatbeh.2008.03.002

116. (Content: I-B-8) A radiotracer with an affinity to orexin is injected during a molecular study. Where is the location the tracer is most likely to accumulate?

A. Arcuate nucleus
B. Lateral hypothalamic area
C. Paraventricular nucleus
D. Melanocortin 3 and 4 receptors

(A) Second-order neurons within the orexigenic pathway, where orexin is found, are located within the lateral hypothalamic area. [Question 8]

Reference: Varela L, Horvath TL. Leptin and insulin pathways in POMC and AgRP neurons that modulate energy balance and glucose homeostasis. EMBO Rep. 2012;13(12):1079-1086. doi:10.1038/embor.2012.174

117. (Content: III-D-2) A mother brings her 17-year-old daughter in for evaluation after recently finding that she has trouble focusing throughout the day. She stays up late and has difficulty falling asleep. The patient was recently started on medication to help with weight loss which she takes daily with lunch. The medication the patient was most likely started on has a mechanism most similar to which of the following?

A. Zonisomide
B. Dulaglutide
C. Diethylpropion
D. Verenacylcine

(C) Phentermine is FDA approved for weight loss in adolescents > 16 years of age or older for a 3-month duration (long-term use is preferred but considered off-label use). Its side effects are similar to stimulants such as diethylpropion, including insomnia. [Questions 105 and 146]

Reference: Phentermine/topiramate ER package insert

118. (Content: III-B-1 and 4) A patient is interested in a low-fat diet due to hypercholesterolemia and a prior myocardial infarction. This diet is sustained for six months. Although the patient denies significant weight loss, he feels better and admits to having more energy. If labs are obtained today, which of the following would likely improve the most?

A. LDL cholesterol
B. HbA1c levels
C. Triglycerides
D. Total cholesterol

(A) In general, low carbohydrate diets have more significant improvements in HDL and TG, whereas fat restriction improves LDL. Improvements in insulin resistance, glucose levels, and HbA1c are only apparent with weight loss in the setting of a low-fat diet but improve independently of weight loss in a carbohydrate-restricted diet. [Question 174]

Reference: Obesity medicine association: Obesity Algorithm (2021)

119. (Content: II-A-4) A 55-year-old female presents to the clinic regarding significant insomnia interfering with her quality of life. She has tried melatonin, sleep hygiene, and cognitive behavioral therapy without success. Zaleplon is prescribed short-term. Which condition is associated with this medication?

    A. Binge eating disorder
    B. Anti-psychotic induced weight gain
    C. Sleep-related eating disorder
    D. Night eating syndrome

(C) Antipsychotics and psychotropic medications (such as sedative-hypnotics) are associated with sleep-related eating disorder, a parasomnia often referred to as "sleep eating." This condition affects 3% of the general population. [Question 87]

Reference: Up To Date: "Disorders of arousal from non-rapid eye movement sleep in adults"

120. (Content: I-B-3) A recent medication has been found to increase adipose tissue that contains significantly more mitochondria. If studied further, this adipose tissue would display what quality?

    A. Mechanically inefficient
    B. Reduces core body temperature
    C. Promotes energy expenditure through shivering
    D. Suppresses metabolic rate proportionately

(A) Brown adipose tissue contains numerous large mitochondria (giving it its brown color), and serves as a warming mechanism for vital organs by uncoupling oxidative phosphorylation, thereby generating heat instead of energy (ATP) via non-shivering thermogenesis. [Question 43]

Reference: Chronic mirabegron treatment increases human brown fat, HDL cholesterol, and insulin sensitivity. O'Mara et al. J Clin Invest. 2020 Jan 21. pii: 131126. doi: 10.1172/JCI131126. [Epub ahead of print]. PMID: 31961826.
Reference: Virtanen et al. NEJM 4/9/2009; 360:1518-1525; DOI: 10.1056/NEJMoa0808949

121. (Content: I-B-1) A patient who has undergone a sleeve gastrectomy is most likely to have which of the following direct neurohormonal responses?

A. Activation of the POMC/CART pathway
B. Inhibition of the NPY/AgRP
C. Decreased activation of the NPY/AgRP
D. Suppression of the POMC/CART pathway

(C) Sleeve gastrectomy, with the removal of up to 80% of the stomach, reduces ghrelin levels, thereby significantly decreasing appetite via decreased activation of the NPY/AgRP orexigenic pathway. [Question 12]

Reference: Ochner CN, Gibson C, Shanik M, Goel V, Geliebter A. Changes in neurohormonal gut peptides following bariatric surgery. Int J Obes (Lond). 2011;35(2):153-166. doi:10.1038/ijo.2010.132

122. (Content: I-B-7) Glucagon-like peptide 1 is secreted by what cell type in the small intestines?

A. I-cells
B. K-cells
C. L-cells
D. S-cells

(C) Cholecystokinin is secreted by I-cells, glucose-dependent insulinotropic peptide by K-cells, and glucagon-like peptide 1, oxyntomodulin, and peptide YY are all secreted by L-cells. [Question 1]

Reference: Miller GD. Appetite Regulation: Hormones, Peptides, and Neurotransmitters and Their Role in Obesity. Am J Lifestyle Med. 2017;13(6):586-601. Published 2017 Jun 23. doi:10.1177/1559827617716376

123. (Content: III-A-1 and 2) A patient returns for a one-month follow-up visit with the dietician. Since the prior visit, the patient has not lost any weight and is frustrated, stating, "I can't lose any weight; I am a failure." Which of the following statements would most effectively assist with weight loss at his next visit?

A. What amount of weight loss would make you feel like you are successful?
B. I know it is frustrating, but I believe in you.
C. Have you been monitoring your caloric intake?
D. What is one thing you can change over the next month?

(D) Motivational interviewing and cognitive-behavioral therapy (CBT) lead to higher patient engagement and ownership while decreasing resistance/barriers and improving overall outcomes. CBT focuses on changing behaviors through cognitive restructuring to reinforce good behaviors and extinguish undesirable ones. One of the components of cognitive-behavioral therapy includes goal setting. [Questions 110 and 127]

Reference: Dalle Grave R, Centis E, Marzocchi R, El Ghoch M, Marchesini G. Major factors for facilitating change in behavioral strategies to reduce obesity. Psychol Res Behav Manag. 2013;6:101-110. Published 2013 Oct 3. doi:10.2147/PRBM.S40460
Reference: Obesity Medicine Association: Obesity Algorithm (2021)

124. (Content: II-D-2) A weight management clinic acquires a duel-energy x-ray absorptiometry (DXA) scan that detects body mass which excludes both essential and nonessential fat. Which of the following terms does this describe?

A. Lean mass
B. Fat-free mass
C. Total body mass
D. Percent body fat

(B) Fat-free mass does not include ANY body fat in its calculation. [Question 69]

Reference: Obesity medicine association: Obesity Algorithm (2021)

125. (Content: II-C-2) A local gym provides screening for cardiovascular risk factors and then provides a customized fitness plan to improve metabolic parameters. In particular, they focus on those with a moderate BMI with abdominal obesity. Which of the following ethnicities and waist circumferences would meet this parameter?

A. Caucasian male: 39 inches (99 cm)
B. Asian male: 31.5 inches (80 cm)
C. Caucasian female: 33 inches (83.3 cm)
D. Asian female: 35 inches (89 cm)

(D) Waist circumference cut-offs of ≥85 cm for men and ≥ 74-80 cm for women is consistent with abdominal obesity in South Asian, Southeast Asian, and East Asian adults. In the U.S. and Canada, waist circumference cut-offs for males are > 102 cm (> 40 in) and for females > 88 cm (> 35 in). [Question 49]

Reference: AACE/ACE Guidelines: AMERICAN ASSOCIATION OF CLINICAL ENDOCRINOLOGISTS AND AMERICAN COLLEGE OF ENDOCRINOLOGY COMPREHENSIVE CLINICAL PRACTICE GUIDELINES FOR MEDICAL CARE OF PATIENTS WITH OBESITY (2016). Recommendation 6-7, and Figure 2.

126. (Content: III-B-1) A 36-year-old female with type II diabetes wants to discuss different dietary patterns. She has a friend that had success with a ketogenic diet, and she was planning to initiate that eating plan on her return from vacation. Which of her medications should be discontinued before starting this diet?

A. Metformin
B. Insulin glargine
C. Dulaglutide
D. Empagliflozin

(D) Extreme caution should be used if a patient is starting a ketogenic diet and is currently taking an SGLT-2 due to the risk of ketoacidosis. [Question 97]

Reference: Obesity medicine association: Obesity Algorithm (2021)

127. (Content: III-F-5c) A 44-year-old male with a history of a recent duodenal switch presents to the emergency department with vomiting and ataxia. If this vitamin deficiency is not corrected, which of the following may be the clinical outcome?

A. Osteoporosis
B. Cardiomyopathy
C. Mucosal bleeding
D. Severe diarrhea

(B) Thiamine (B₁) deficiency can lead to wet beriberi (high-output congestive heart failure including cardiomegaly, cardiomyopathy, peripheral edema, and tachycardia), dry beriberi (symmetric peripheral polyneuropathy affecting sensory and motor function) mostly affecting the distal extremities, Wernicke's encephalopathy (ataxia, nystagmus, ophthalmoplegia, and confusion; considered reversible), and Korsakoff syndrome (irreversible, a chronic neurological condition characterized by impaired short-term memory and confabulation). [Question 104]

Reference: Up to Date: "Overview of water-soluble vitamins"

128. (Content: III-A-2) Which of the following is the best example of a SMART goal?

A. Lose weight by the end of the month by walking daily
B. Continue to avoid soda intake for the year
C. Reduce eating fast food to only once weekly
D. Hire a trainer to develop a weekly exercise plan

*(C) A **SMART** goal is an acronym for setting a quality and challenging goal. It stands for **S**pecific, **M**easurable, **A**chievable, **R**elevant, and **T**imed. [Question 214]*

Reference: Bovend'Eerdt TJ, Botell RE, Wade DT. Writing SMART rehabilitation goals and achieving goal attainment scaling: a practical guide [published correction appears in Clin Rehabil. 2010 Apr;24(4):382]. Clin Rehabil. 2009;23(4):352-361. doi:10.1177/0269215508101741

129. (Content: II-D-3a) A 42-year-old male with class II obesity presents to the clinic for abnormalities on laboratory examination of the liver. In particular, his AST and ALT are elevated. He denies alcohol use. A liver biopsy is completed and shows hepatosteatitis. Which of the following is consistent with this diagnosis?

    A. Fatty liver with the absence of inflammation
    B. Hepatic injury present with irreversible nodules
    C. Potential improvement from metformin use
    D. Hepatic inflammation without cirrhosis

(D) Metabolic-associated fatty liver disease (MAFLD) encompasses a spectrum of conditions, including hepatosteatosis (fatty liver), hepatosteatitis (fatty liver with inflammation), and metabolic-associated steatohepatitis (presence of > 5% hepatic fat with inflammation and hepatocyte injury, +/- cirrhosis). Note that MAFLD has replaced the non-alcoholic (NAFLD) nomenclature. [Question 63]

Reference: AACE/ACE Guidelines: AMERICAN ASSOCIATION OF CLINICAL ENDOCRINOLOGISTS AND AMERICAN COLLEGE OF ENDOCRINOLOGY COMPREHENSIVE CLINICAL PRACTICE GUIDELINES FOR MEDICAL CARE OF PATIENTS WITH OBESITY (2016). Recommendation 16.
Reference: Obesity medicine association: Obesity Algorithm (2021)

130. (Content: II-D-3a) An asymptomatic patient undergoes a sleep study before bariatric surgery. During the study, she averaged ten episodes per 1 hour of oxygen desaturation from 98% to 93%, accompanied by periods of shallow breathing. Which finding does this most likely represent?

    A. Apnea
    B. Obstructive sleep apnea
    C. Central sleep apnea
    D. Hypopnea

(D) Apnea involves respiratory pauses that last ≥ 10 seconds, whereas hypopnea includes shallow breathing leading to oxygen desaturation of 4%. [Question 52]

Reference: Up To Date: "Clinical manifestations and diagnosis of OSA in adults"

131. (Content: III-D-5) Which of the following supplements is most closely associated with hepatic injury?

A. Green tea extract
B. Chitosan
C. Raspberry extract
D. Ephedra

(A) Green tea extract is an important and well-known cause of hepatic injury, along with the more common side effects similar to caffeine excess. [Question 200]

Reference: Obesity medicine association: Obesity Algorithm (2021)

132. (Content: I-A-3) A pediatric male patient presents to an obesity specialist to be evaluated for secondary causes of obesity. He has a history of seizures and developmental delay. On exam, he is noted to have more prominent earlobes and gynecomastia with underdeveloped genitals. What is the most likely syndrome?

A. Borgeson-Forssman-Lehmann
B. Cohen
C. Prader-Willi
D. Bardet-Biedl

(A) Borgeson-Forssman-Lehmann syndrome is x-linked (males affected) and associated with seizures, large earlobes, short toes, gynecomastia, excess weight, intellectual disability, and small genitals. [Question 23]

Reference: Up To Date: "Genetic contribution and pathophysiology of obesity."

133. (Content: I-A-5) The highest predictor of childhood obesity is in infants with which of the following characteristics?

A. Born one week past the due date
B. On-demand breast-fed infants
C. Marijuana use during pregnancy
D. **Both parents have BMI ≥35 kg/m²**

(D) Many correlations between childhood obesity related to maternal and early infancy environments have been discovered (i.e., epigenetics). Notably, if one parent has obesity, there is a 3x risk of developing obesity. If both parents have obesity, there is a 10x risk for the child. [Question 26]

Reference: Obesity medicine association: Pediatric Obesity Algorithm (2020-2022)

134. (Content: III-D-6) A patient reads about a home remedy for weight loss that includes high doses of psyllium. The patient tolerates it initially but states it is causing gastrointestinal distress. Which mechanism is best attributed to her weight loss treatment?

A. Increased energy expenditure
B. Decreased dietary fat absorption
C. Increased fat oxidation
D. **Improved satiety**

(D) Supplements marketed to improve satiety include guar gum, psyllium, and prebiotic fiber. [Question 109]

Reference: Up to Date: "Overview of herbal medicine and dietary supplements"

135. (Content: III-F-3) A 17-year-old female underwent a Roux-en-Y gastric bypass. Twenty-four hours postoperatively, she complains of increasing abdominal and chest pain. The heart rate is elevated and blood counts reveal an elevated leukocyte count. Which of the following is the most likely cause of this patient's primary pathology causing her symptoms?

    A. Pulmonary arteries
    B. Pulmonary parenchyma
    C. Gastrointestinal anastomosis site
    D. Peritoneal and diaphragmatic surfaces

(C) Anastomotic leaks usually occur within the first few days of surgery. It more commonly occurs at the gastrojejunostomy anastomosis and presents as fever, worsening abdominal or chest pain, tachycardia, and leukocytosis. *[Question 120]*

Reference: Obesity medicine association: Obesity Algorithm (2021)

136. (Content: I-D-3) A study is being performed to determine the prevalence of vitamin deficiencies in those with obesity. One hundred participants undergo vitamin laboratory analysis. Which is the most prevalent deficiency in this population?

    A. Thiamine
    B. Iron
    C. Vitamin D
    D. Folate

(C) The prevalence of vitamin D (a fat-soluble vitamin) deficiency in obesity is greater than 30% due to body dilution, as skin surface area is not proportionate to patient volume. [Question 35]

Reference: Dietary Calcium Intake and Obesity; Sarina Schrager. The Journal of the American Board of Family Practice May 2005, 18 (3) 205-210; DOI: https://doi.org/10.3122/jabfm.18.3.205

137. (Content: I-A-4) A 9-year-old female presents with her parents to a pediatric weight management clinic. The patient's height, weight, and BMI have increased significantly over the past few years. The patient has developed breast buds. Which of the following is the most likely etiology?

    A. Normal prepubertal development
    B. Hypothyroidism
    C. Increased caloric intake
    D. Underlying genetic condition

(C) Excessive caloric intake and precocious puberty would cause accelerated linear bone growth proportionate to weight gain. Although syndromic obesity could cause decreased bone growth, excessive weight gain usually occurs earlier and is accompanied by developmental delay. Those with endocrinopathies such as hypercortisolism or thyroid disorders will significantly increase weight compared to height. [Question 21]

Reference: Obesity medicine association: Pediatric Obesity Algorithm (2020-2022)

138. (Content: III-F-1) Which of the following best describes the anatomical differences between a duodenal switch (DS) and a Roux-en-Y gastric bypass (RYGB)?

    A. DS has a shorter common channel
    B. RYGB removes a more significant portion of the stomach
    C. The biliopancreatic loop in RYGB is primarily made from the jejunum
    D. The digestive loop in the DS is most prone to small bacterial intestinal overgrowth

(A) The DS is a malabsorptive procedure in which the stomach is made into a tubular pouch (4-8 oz), and a surgical "duodenal switch" delays the combination of the food (digestive loop) with the digestive enzymes (biliopancreatic loop), until 75-150 cm before the large intestine (common channel). This common channel is much shorter than in a RYGB. [Question 171]

Reference: Up to Date: "Bariatric procedures for the management of severe obesity: Descriptions"

139. (Content: II-B-4) A patient was diagnosed with night eating syndrome and underwent cognitive behavioral therapy. Although improvements are noted in eating behaviors, the patient is interested in pharmacotherapy. Which of the following is the most efficacious option?

A. Phentermine
B. Metformin
C. Sertraline
D. Bupropion

(C) Treatment for night eating syndrome (NES) is focused on encouraging regular meal consumption earlier in the daytime, with increased protein intake being very effective. Cognitive-behavioral therapy can help with many eating disorders, including NES. Pharmacotherapy may be considered, including selective serotonin reuptake inhibitors, with a high response rate to sertraline. [Question 85]

Reference: Allison KC, Tarves EP. Treatment of night eating syndrome. Psychiatr Clin North Am. 2011;34(4):785–796. doi:10.1016/j.psc.2011.08.002

140. (Content: II-D-3b) A 26-year-old female presents for a gynecologic evaluation after being evaluated in the emergency department for pelvic pain. A pregnancy test was negative and an ultrasound revealed multiple bilateral ovarian cysts. Which of the following would most likely be decreased in this patient?

A. Sex hormone binding globulin
B. Luteinizing: follicular stimulating hormone ratio
C. Androgens
D. Prolactin

(A) Sex hormone binding globulin is decreased in patients with obesity and those with polycystic ovarian syndrome. [Questions 79 and 91]

Reference: Up to Date: "Diagnosis of polycystic ovary syndrome in adults"
Reference: Zhu JL, Chen Z, Feng WJ, Long SL, Mo ZC. Sex hormone-binding globulin and polycystic ovary syndrome. Clin Chim Acta. 2019 Dec;499:142-148. doi: 10.1016/j.cca.2019.09.010. Epub 2019 Sep 13. PMID: 31525346.
Reference: Cooper LA, Page ST, Amory JK, Anawalt BD, Matsumoto AM. The association of obesity with sex hormone-binding globulin is stronger than the association with ageing--implications for the interpretation of total testosterone measurements. Clin Endocrinol (Oxf). 2015 Dec;83(6):828-33. doi: 10.1111/cen.12768. Epub 2015 May 11. PMID: 25777143; PMCID: PMC4782930.

141. (Content: III-G-7) A female patient with pre-diabetes presents to her primary care physician to discuss the initiation of metformin. According to the American Diabetes Association, in what scenario should metformin be considered for this patient?

A. Age greater than 45 years old
B. **History of gestational diabetes**
C. A body mass index of 30 kg/m^2
D. A strong family history of diabetes

(B) Pharmacotherapy with metformin should be considered in those with prediabetes (HbA1c 5.7%- 6.4%), especially if the patient is < 60 years old, has a BMI ≥ 35 kg/m^2, or in females with a history of gestational diabetes. Metformin reduces the risk of progression to diabetes by 31%. [Question 205]

Reference: American Diabetes Association: Standards of Medical Care in Diabetes—2020 Abridged for Primary Care Providers; Clinical Diabetes 2020 Jan; 38(1): 10-38. https://doi.org/10.2337/cd20-as01
Reference: Knowler WC, Barrett-Connor E, Fowler SE, et al. Reduction in the incidence of type 2 diabetes with lifestyle intervention or metformin. N Engl J Med. 2002;346(6):393-403. doi:10.1056/NEJMoa012512

142. (Content: III-C-1) An exercise prescription is written for a patient following an initial consultation with an obesity medicine specialist. Regarding the acronym 'FITTE' used to write the script, what does the 'I' stand for?

A. Instructions
B. Intervals
C. Interests
D. **Intensity**

*(D) An exercise prescription should be very specific and include **f**requency, **i**ntensity, **t**ime, **t**ype, and **e**njoyment (FITTE). [Question 155]*

Reference: Physical Activity Guidelines for Americans: 2nd Edition: https://health.gov/sites/default/files/2019-09/Physical_Activity_Guidelines_2nd_edition.pdf

143. (Content: III-A-1) A psychiatrist meets with a patient for a consultation before a sleeve gastrectomy. She utilizes 'evoking,' a key process of motivational interviewing. What phrase is most consistent with that key process?

  A. **What is your most significant motivation to improve your health?**
  B. I want you to know that everything you tell me today is confidential.
  C. Let's write out some short-term and long-term weight goals.
  D. It seems like you struggle to eat healthily while at work. Tell me more about this.

(A) Evoking is a key process of motivational interviewing, along with focusing, planning, and engagement. Evoking involves discovering the patient's interest and motivation to change and using these to reach their goals. [Question 186]

Reference: Obesity medicine association: Obesity Algorithm (2021)

144. (Content: III-F-4) Which would be a beneficial reason for allowing a pre-operative gastric bypass patient to consume carbohydrates up to 2 hours before anesthesia induction?

  A. Prevent post-operative nausea
  B. Allow for earlier detection of extraluminal leaks
  C. **Improve insulin resistance**
  D. Reduce the need for diphenoxylate postoperatively

(C) Preoperative enhanced recovery after bariatric surgery (ERABS) clinical pathways should be implemented in all patients undergoing bariatric surgery to improve postoperative outcomes. This includes allowing the patient to have oral nutrition with carbohydrates up to 2 hours preoperatively to decrease insulin resistance, decrease protein catabolism, reduce hospital length of stay, and experience a faster return of bowel function. [Question 111]

Reference: AACE/TOS/ASMBS/OMA/ASA 2019 Guidelines: CLINICAL PRACTICE GUIDELINES FOR THE PERIOPERATIVE NUTRITION, METABOLIC, AND NONSURGICAL SUPPORT OF PATIENTS UNDERGOING BARIATRIC PROCEDURES – 2019 UPDATE. Recommendation 34, 35, 36, 40. Table 8.

145. (Content: III-H-1 and 3 and III-F-6) Which of the following pediatric patients should start the 4-tiered approach for managing pediatric obesity, compared to those who can continue with prevention of obesity management only?

    A. A patient with a BMI in the 80th percentile with type 1 diabetes
    B. A patient with a BMI in the 85th percentile with tonsillar hypertrophy
    C. A patient with a BMI in the 90th percentile with Bartter syndrome
    D. A patient with a BMI in the 95th percentile with no comorbidities

(D) Pediatric patients recommended to start the 4-tiered approach for management of pediatric obesity include those with a BMI ≥ 95th percentile or those with a BMI 85th-94th percentile with obesity-related health risks (such as fatty liver disease, sleep apnea, hypertension, type 2 diabetes, etc.). [Questions 130 and 197]

Reference: Expert Committee Recommendations Regarding the Prevention, Assessment, and Treatment of Child and Adolescent Overweight and Obesity: Summary Report. Sarah E. Barlow. Pediatrics Dec 2007, 120 (Supplement 4) S164-S192; DOI: 10.1542/peds.2007-2329C

146. (Content: IV-C) The American College of Cardiology recommends which individuals undergo a stress electrocardiogram test if planning to start a vigorous exercise plan?

    A. Women > 50 years old who are asymptomatic
    B. Anyone over the age of 55 years with diabetes
    C. Deconditioned males over the age of 35 years old
    D. In those with a family history of cardiomyopathy

(A) The American College of Cardiology has recommended performing stress electrocardiograms in high-risk individuals before starting exercise programs. These include asymptomatic individuals who have multiple cardiac risk factors or men > 40 years old and women > 50 years old who plan to start vigorous exercise. [Question 219]

Reference: Screening for cardiovascular disease risk with electrocardiogram: USPTF Recommendation. https://www.acc.org/latest-in-cardiology/journal-scans/2018/06/14/14/41/screening-for-cardiovascular-disease-risk-with-ecg

147. (Content: II-E, II-F, and II-A-3) A clinic has created a limited program to capture and work closely with those at risk for obesity-related complications. This will include follow-up with a dietician and a trainer to provide a customized plan. Initially, they want to limit this to patients with a BMI of ≥ 30 kg/m^2. Of these patients, which ones should receive priority?

A. Males with a waist circumference of 99 cm (39 inches)
B. Patients with an Edmonton Obesity Staging System stage 2
C. Patients with prediabetes or mild osteoarthritis
D. Those with a family history of coronary artery disease

(B) The Edmonton Obesity Staging System provides better insight into the patient's long-term impact of obesity and may help determine the level of appropriate treatment (along with established metrics). It is used to categorize patients based on the severity of obesity-related comorbidities, psychologic symptoms, and functional limitations rather than focusing strictly on anthropometric measurements. [Questions 68 and 84]

Reference: Using the Edmonton obesity staging system to predict mortality in a population-representative cohort of people with overweight and obesity. Raj S. Padwal, Nicholas M. Pajewski, David B. Allison and Arya M. Sharma. CMAJ October 04, 2011 183 (14) E1059-E1066; DOI: https://doi.org/10.1503/cmaj.110387
Reference: "Assessment of obesity beyond body mass index to determine benefit of treatment." E. T. Aasheim, S. J. B. Aylwin, S. T. Radhakrishnan, A. S. Sood, A. Jovanovic, T. Olbers, C. W. le Roux, First published: 05 July 2011 https://doi.org/10.1111/j.1758-8111.2011.00017.x

148. (Content: II-C-7) A 14-year-old male presents to clinic. His body mass index of 36 kg/m^2 is in the 99th percentile range based on age and gender. Which of the following most accurately describes his weight categorization?

A. Overweight
B. Obesity class I
C. Obesity class II
D. Obesity class III

(C) Obesity class II, for those ages 2-19, is defined as > 120% of the 95th percentile based on age and gender, or a BMI of ≥ 35 kg/m^2. [Question 59]

Reference: Obesity medicine association: Pediatric Obesity Algorithm (2020-2022)

149. (Content: III-G-6) The Centers for Disease Control and Prevention recognizes which of the following malignancies has a direct correlation with excess weight?

A. Testicular cancer
B. **Colorectal cancer**
C. Cholangiocarcinoma
D. Chronic Leukemia

(B) The CDC recognizes 13 malignancies that are increased in the setting of having excess weight (BMI ≥ 25kg/m²). This is thought to be from the increased inflammatory cytokines, sex hormones, and insulin resistance associated with excess adipose tissue. This includes breast (post-menopausal), colorectal, esophageal (adenocarcinoma), gallbladder, stomach (upper), kidneys, liver, pancreas, ovaries, multiple myeloma, meningioma, uterus, and thyroid malignancies. [Question 183]

Reference: CDC: Obesity and Cancer.
Reference: American Cancer Society: Does Body Weight Affect Cancer Risk?

150. (Content: III-F-3) A 54-year-old patient is admitted to the hospital with an elevated D-lactose level in the setting of encephalopathy and ataxia. The patient underwent a successful Roux-en-Y gastric bypass three years prior. Which of the following likely explains these findings?

A. Acute alcohol intoxication
B. **Small intestinal bowel overgrowth**
C. Thiamine deficiency
D. A surgical emergency

(B) Patients with small intestinal bacterial overgrowth (SIBO) often present with bloating, abdominal pain, and watery diarrhea. It can also cause the production of toxins such as D-lactic acidosis, which may cause neurologic changes such as confusion, ataxia, and seizures. [Question 125]

Reference: Up to Date: "Small intestinal bacterial overgrowth: Clinical manifestations and diagnosis"
Reference: Up to Date: "Small intestinal bacterial overgrowth: Etiology and pathogenesis"

151. (Content: I-A-5) A mother presents to her gynecologist and requests recommendations to ensure her infant doesn't develop obesity. She has struggled with weight throughout her adult life and wants to ensure her newborn has the best chance to maintain good health. What advice is most appropriate at this time?

A. Feed the infant a lower protein diet
B. Reduce carbohydrate-rich foods during pregnancy
C. Avoid breastfeeding the infant due to the high sugar content
D. Early complimentary feedings in an infant reduce the risk of obesity

(B) Several perinatal risk factors influence weight gain in infants. Feeding habits such as high protein intake, early complementary feedings, and added sugars increase the risk of increased toddler weight. In females who have excess weight before pregnancy and develop gestational diabetes (i.e., insulin resistance), childhood obesity rates are the highest. Thus parental education, strict insulin control, role-modeling healthy habits, and reducing high-density and carbohydrate-rich foods should be emphasized. [Question 39]

Reference: Obesity medicine association: Pediatric Obesity Algorithm (2020-2022)

152. (Content: III-D-8) A 51-year-old has neuropathy due to amyloidosis, as well as sleep-onset insomnia. The patient's BMI is 36 kg/m^2. Which medication would be most appropriate to start at this time?

A. Amitriptyline
B. Imipramine
C. Nortriptyline
D. Mirtazepine

(C) Tricyclic antidepressants (TCA) can treat both insomnia and neuropathic pain. Of the TCA medications, desipramine and nortriptyline are the most weight-neutral options. [Question 204]

Reference: Obesity medicine association: Obesity Algorithm (2021)

153. (Content: II-C-6) A 33-year-old male presents for his 4-month post-Roux-en-Y gastric bypass surgery follow-up visit. He has not tolerated a solid diet and has been non-adherent with his medications. He is complaining of diarrhea which has not improved despite loperamide. On physical examination, a rash is noted on his lower extremities. Which finding would most likely occur if this particular vitamin deficiency is not corrected?

A. **Memory issues**
B. Lower extremity edema
C. Macrocytic anemia
D. Neuropathy

(A) Niacin deficiency (B₃), also known as pellagra, can cause symptoms ranging from dermatitis, diarrhea, dementia, and eventually death. [Question 65]

Reference: Up to Date: "Overview of water-soluble vitamins"

154. (Content: II-A-3) Which of the following is a characteristic commonly included in the diagnosis of metabolic syndrome?

A. Liver function tests
B. Low-density lipoprotein
C. Body mass index
D. **Fasting plasma glucose**

(D) Diagnostic criteria for metabolic syndrome are based on the presence of at least 3 of the following: abdominal obesity, hypertriglyceridemia, low serum high-density lipoprotein (HDL) cholesterol, elevated blood pressure, and increased fasting plasma glucose. [Question 60]

Reference: Up to Date: "Metabolic syndrome (insulin resistance syndrome or syndrome X)"

155. (Content: III-G-1) An elderly male with class I obesity is seen by a nursing home physician after being hospitalized for four weeks with COVID pneumonia. He does not have the strength to stand for longer than 1 minute and cannot perform repetitive tasks like raising his hands. His weight is now similar to his pre-covid diagnosis. What diagnosis most accurately reflects his findings?

A. Steroid-induced polymyositis
B. Sarcopenic obesity
C. Normal changes with aging
D. Malnourishment

(B) Patients can increase their weight, without increasing muscle mass, by adding adipose tissue (i.e., sarcopenic obesity). Weight loss in the setting of malnutrition or debility often reduces lean body mass, including muscle mass, which is disproportionately more difficult to regain. *[Question 128]*

Reference: Morley JE. Treatment of sarcopenia: the road to the future. J Cachexia Sarcopenia Muscle. 2018;9(7):1196-1199. doi:10.1002/jcsm.12386

156. (Content: I-B-7.) Which of the following anorexigenic intestinal hormones is secreted by the small intestines to slow gastric emptying and aid in fat digestion?

A. Peptide YY
B. Glucagon-like peptide 1
C. Oxyntomodulin
D. Cholecystokinin

(D) Cholecystokinin is secreted by the duodenum and jejunum (I-cells) and stimulates gallbladder contraction, slows gastric emptying, and reduces appetite. [Question 1]

Reference: Miller GD. Appetite Regulation: Hormones, Peptides, and Neurotransmitters and Their Role in Obesity. Am J Lifestyle Med. 2017;13(6):586-601. Published 2017 Jun 23. doi:10.1177/1559827617716376

157. (Content: III-A-1) A structural framework is utilized when performing motivational interviewing on a patient attempting to lose weight. The OARS framework is used. What does the "O" stand for in this acronym?

- A. Outside influences
- B. Obstructions that require a change
- **C. Open-ended questions**
- D. Opportunities to change

*(C) **OARS** is an acronym commonly used as a motivational interviewing skill that leads to higher patient engagement and ownership while decreasing resistance/barriers and improving overall outcomes. It stands for **O**pen-ended questions, **A**ffirmations, **R**eflection, and **S**ummarize. [Question 110]*

Reference: Obesity Medicine Association: Obesity Algorithm (2021)

158. (Content: III-F-1 and 2) A 63-year-old male presents to a metabolic and bariatric surgical clinic to discuss weight loss options. He has read about the TransPyloric Shuttle® and would like to know if he is a candidate for this device placement. Which of the following is a contraindication to this device?

- A. History of colectomy due to colon cancer
- **B. Taking anticoagulation for atrial fibrillation**
- C. Treatment for H. Pylori within the past six months
- D. Prior history of NSAID-induced gastric ulcer

(B) Contraindications of the TransPyloric Shuttle® include altered upper gastrointestinal anatomy such as a stricture or prior surgery, esophageal varices, current erosions, ulcerations, untreated H. pylori infections, current gastritis, pregnancy, and coagulopathy (including being on anticoagulation). [Question 175]

Reference: FDA- TransPyloric Shuttle/TransPyloric Shuttle Delivery Device - P180024

159. (Content: III-F-5c) A patient underwent the most common bariatric surgery and is doing well afterward. Which of the following is most likely decreased in this patient post-operatively?

    A. Cells directly producing Ghrelin
    B. Risk of acid reflux
    C. Glucagon-like peptide 1 secretion
    D. Vitamin absorptive capacity

(A) Sleeve gastrectomy is the most common bariatric procedure performed worldwide. Removing 80% of the stomach also removes gastric parietal cells (which make intrinsic factor and ghrelin). [Question 118]

Reference: GVL.png. (2018, November 19). Wikimedia Commons, the free media repository. Retrieved 5/3/2020 from https://commons.wikimedia.org/w/index.php?title=File:GVL.png&oldid=328277494.
[1]Reference: McTigue KM, Wellman R, Nauman E, et al. Comparing the 5-Year Diabetes Outcomes of Sleeve Gastrectomy and Gastric Bypass: The National Patient-Centered Clinical Research Network (PCORNet) Bariatric Study. JAMA Surg. Published online March 04, 2020. doi:10.1001/jamasurg.2020.0087

160. (Content: I-C-1) The federal government approves a graduated budgetary allowance to the states with the highest rates of obesity prevalence. Which state would likely receive the most significant financial influx?

    A. California
    B. Colorado
    C. West Virginia
    D. Florida

(C) States in the Southeast tend to have the highest rates of obesity. Mississippi (40.8%) and West Virginia (39.7%) have the two highest rates of obesity in the United States. [Question 16]

Reference: https://www.cdc.gov/nccdphp/dnpao/data-trends-maps/index.html

161. (Content: III-D-4) A maximum dose of phentermine/topiramate ER (Qsymia®) would include what dose range for the topiramate ER?

A. 0-25 mg
B. 25-50 mg
C. 50-75 mg
D. 75-100 mg

(D) The maximum dose of phentermine/topiramate ER (Qsymia®) is 15/92 mg daily. If weight loss is less than 5% of total body weight at maximum dose, the medication should be discontinued and alternatives trialed. [Question 158]

Reference: Phentermine/topiramate ER package insert

162. (Content: I-B-4) A patient saw the term "adiposopathy" on their chart and was unsure how this related to her comorbidities of obesity. Which of the following conditions is this likely referring to?

A. Atherosclerosis of the carotid artery
B. Heart failure with a preserved ejection fraction
C. Osteoarthritis of the knees
D. Obstructive sleep apnea

(A) Both fat mass disease and sick fat disease (adiposopathy) are pathogenic components of obesity. Fat mass refers to the mechanical forces acting on the body, whereas sick fat disease refers to the inflammatory/hormonal effects. [Question 18]

Reference: De Lorenzo A, Soldati L, Sarlo F, Calvani M, Di Lorenzo N, Di Renzo L. New obesity classification criteria as a tool for bariatric surgery indication. World J Gastroenterol. 2016;22(2):681-703. doi:10.3748/wjg.v22.i2.681

163. (Content: III-F-4) A 33-year-old female would like to undergo bariatric surgery to improve her health and reduce her risk of future pregnancy complications. She has been diagnosed with polycystic ovarian syndrome, which has impaired her ability to get pregnant. She is hoping that with substantial weight loss, she will be more likely to become pregnant. What is the minimum recommended time frame after surgery she should be instructed to avoid pregnancy?

 A. 3 months
 B. 6 months
 C. 9 months
 D. 12 months

(D) In women undergoing bariatric surgery, pregnancy should be avoided preoperatively and 12-18 months postoperatively. [Question 192]

Reference: AACE/TOS/ASMBS/OMA/ASA 2019 Guidelines: CLINICAL PRACTICE GUIDELINES FOR THE PERIOPERATIVE NUTRITION, METABOLIC, AND NONSURGICAL SUPPORT OF PATIENTS UNDERGOING BARIATRIC PROCEDURES – 2019 UPDATE. Recommendation 14, 17, 18, 23

164. (Content: II-D-2) A patient undergoes a dual-energy x-ray absorptiometry test to determine his body fat percentage. Which of the following best reflects this testing modality?

 A. It is considered the gold standard
 B. Any BMI can undergo this testing
 C. It is associated with significant radiation exposure
 D. It is inaccurate if the patient is dehydrated

(A) A dual-energy x-ray absorptiometry is accurate (although it may not accommodate those with extreme BMI), relatively inexpensive, and considered the gold standard. [Question 50]

Reference: Obesity Medicine Association: Obesity Algorithm (2021)

165. (Content: II-C-3 and I-B-4) A 12-year-old male presents to his pediatrician with an abnormal gait. His parents have noticed it more during the pandemic when they state his weight has increased due to less physical activity. Examination reveals bowing of the tibia. His mother states there are no dietary restrictions. Which of the following is the most likely etiology of his presentation?

    A. Ricket's
    B. Legg-Calve-Perthes disease
    C. Slipped capital femoral epiphysis
    D. Blount disease

(D) Blount disease is bowing of the tibia (varus) and can be seen in children with obesity. In contrast, slipped capital femoral epiphysis presents with a new-onset unilateral limp and external rotation (i.e., resistance to internal rotation) due to an unstable proximal femur growth plate. [Question 74]

Reference: Up to Date: Evaluation and Management of Slipped Capital Femoral Epiphysis (SCFE)

166. (Content: II-C-3) A 39-year-old female presents to a family medicine physician frustrated by her inability to lose weight over the past six months. Despite increased exercise and improved eating habits, she feels more tired and gained approximately 15 lbs (6.8kg) over the same time frame. Which skin finding would most likely be seen on a physical exam?

    A. Widened abdominal striae
    B. Xanthelasmas
    C. Acne
    D. Dry and cracked skin

(D) Skin findings associated with hypothyroidism include dry and cracked skin, thinning of eyebrows, and periorbital edema. [Question 82]

Reference: Up to Date: "Overweight and obesity in adults: Health consequences"

167. (Content: I-D-2) Where is the location of vitamin B_{12} absorption within the gastrointestinal tract?

    A. Gastric fundus
    B. Proximal small intestines
    C. Distal small intestines
    D. Colon

(C) Vitamin B_{12} is absorbed in the terminal ileum (distal small intestines), with the co-factor intrinsic factor produced by parietal cells in the stomach. [Questions 27 and 33]

Reference: Up to Date: "Causes and pathophysiology of vitamin B_{12} and folate deficiencies"
Reference: Up to Date: "Bariatric surgery: Postoperative nutritional management"

168. (Content: I-A-5) The consequences of maternal obesity and the intrauterine environment in which a fetus develops affect which of the following?

    A. Genetic mutations
    B. Mitochondrial deletions
    C. DNA expression
    D. Recessive inheritance

(C) The consequences of maternal obesity and the intrauterine environment affect the developing fetus's brain via epigenetics. The term epigenetics refers to modifying genetic expression (not genetic mutations), often in the setting of inheritable changes. [Question 5]

Reference: Assessing the fetal effects of maternal obesity via transcriptomic analysis of cord blood: a prospective case–control study. AG Edlow L Hui HC Wick I Fried DW Bianchi. First published: 29 December 2015

169. (Content: II-D-1) Out of 1000 kcal utilized throughout a day in a resting individual, how many calories would the skeletal muscles consume?

A. 50 kcal
B. 100 kcal
C. 150 kcal
D. 200 kcal

(D) Skeletal muscle and the liver comprise the most substantial portion of the components that make up resting metabolic rate (RMR), accounting for 20% of RMR each. [Question 86]

Reference: Reference: Obesity medicine association: Obesity Algorithm (2021)

170. (Content: III-F-5b) A 61-year-old female who underwent a biliopancreatic diversion with duodenal switch six years prior returns for her annual follow-up appointment. She underwent a dual-energy x-ray absorptiometry and was found to have a T score of -2.6 (reference range: between +1 and -1). She had normal vitamin levels and an unremarkable complete metabolic panel. Which of the following is recommended at this time?

A. Weekly oral alendronate
B. Daily oral alendronate
C. Intravenous zoledronic acid annually
D. One-time subcutaneous denosumab injection

(C) In post-bariatric surgery patients (especially malabsorptive procedures), non-oral antiresorptive agents (intravenous bisphosphonates or subcutaneous denosumab) should be considered in those with osteoporosis who have had vitamin D and calcium levels normalized. This is due to the risk of anastomotic ulceration and diminished absorption with oral formulations. Denosumab has a risk of bone resorption and increased risk of fracture once therapy is discontinued or interrupted, so it should be continued long term or a bisphosphonate should be initiated after stopping therapy. [Question 163]

Reference: AACE/TOS/ASMBS/OMA/ASA 2019 Guidelines: CLINICAL PRACTICE GUIDELINES FOR THE PERIOPERATIVE NUTRITION, METABOLIC, AND NONSURGICAL SUPPORT OF PATIENTS UNDERGOING BARIATRIC PROCEDURES – 2019 UPDATE. Recommendation 53, 54, 55, Table 12

171. (Content: I-C-2) In those aged 2-19 years old, which subset has the highest prevalence rates of obesity?

A. Those with the highest income
B. Caucasian females
C. Asian males
D. Middle-income families

(D) Obesity affects nearly 20% of all children aged 2-19. The prevalence is highest in those with the lowest (18.9%) and middle income (19.9%), likely explained by the increased cost of healthy food and the lack of grocery stores in lower-income neighborhoods. [Question 10]

Reference: CDC: https://www.cdc.gov/obesity/data/childhood.html#Prevalence

172. (Content: III-E) A local supermarket is advertising a new dietary supplement they just started selling. Which of the following describes this substance most accurately?

A. It is considered safe according to the FDA
B. It can be marketed to prevent but not cure diseases
C. It is considered a food, not a drug
D. It has positive effects beyond basic nutrition

(C) A dietary supplement is a substance taken in addition to dietary intake and is not approved by the FDA because they are considered a food, not a drug. [Question 131]

Reference: Obesity medicine association: Obesity Algorithm (2021)

173. (Content: II-A-1) A 51-year-old female presents to a smoking cessation clinic and is prescribed bupropion. Five days later, she is brought to the emergency department by ambulance with convulsive seizures. Which of the following was likely not addressed at the time of medication initiation?

A. Concurrent marijuana use
B. Parotid gland enlargement on exam
C. Current prescription of sertraline
D. Family history of a cranial neoplasm

(B) Bupropion is contraindicated in eating disorders (i.e., bulimia), epilepsy, or other conditions that lower the seizure threshold. Physical exam findings concerning for bulimia include Russell's sign (callouses or cuts on the knuckles due to repetitive self-induced vomiting) and parotid gland enlargement. [Question 77]

Reference: Up To Date: "Eating disorders: Overview of prevention and treatment"

174. (Content II-C-1) An 18-year-old returns from college after her first semester. Her body mass index (BMI) 6 months ago was 29 kg/m^2. However, with her lack of physical activity and increased caloric intake, her BMI has now increased by 2 kg/m^2. Which of the following would best classify her new BMI?

A. Normal weight
B. Overweight
C. Class I obesity
D. Class II obesity

(C) Class 1 obesity is defined as a body mass index between 30-34.9 kg/m^2. [Question 93]

Reference: AACE/ACE Guidelines: AMERICAN ASSOCIATION OF CLINICAL ENDOCRINOLOGISTS AND AMERICAN COLLEGE OF ENDOCRINOLOGY COMPREHENSIVE CLINICAL PRACTICE GUIDELINES FOR MEDICAL CARE OF PATIENTS WITH OBESITY (2016)

175. (Content: I-A-3) Two adolescent patients are seen in a tertiary weight management facility. One has a leptin receptor gene defect, and the other has melanocortin 4 receptor deficiency. What will be the most noticeable difference between these two patients?

A. **Height**
B. Skin pallor
C. Blood pressure
D. Intellectual ability

(A) MC4R mediates most of the anorectic effects of leptin; therefore, a deficiency leads to early-onset obesity via leptin resistance. Interestingly, leptin is also independently involved in linear bone growth, with increased levels causing tall stature in MC4R deficiency. Those with leptin receptor gene defects do not have tall stature. [Question 2]

Reference: Up To Date: "Genetic contribution and pathophysiology of obesity"

176. (Content: III-F-3) The mechanism and effect behind dumping syndrome after a patient undergoes a Roux-en-Y gastric bypass is best described by which of the following statements?

A. High protein osmotic gradient causes rapid gut transit time
B. **Exaggerated insulin secretion leads to hypoglycemia**
C. Large carbohydrate loads cause increased bacterial gas production
D. The bypassed pylorus is unable to regulate the rate of acidotic gastric contents

(B) High carbohydrate loads can rapidly empty into the small bowel as the pyloric mechanism is bypassed after a RYGB. Although the rapid glucose absorption initially leads to hyperglycemia, the subsequent exaggerated insulin release can cause symptomatic hypoglycemia. [Question 119]

Reference: Up to Date: "Laparoscopic Roux-en-Y gastric bypass"

177. (Content: I-B-5) During an evaluation for weight loss surgery, a dietician estimates the patient's total energy expenditure (TEE). The dietician tells the patient the TEE may be under-evaluated due to non-exercise activity thermogenesis. What is the dietician referring to?

A. Calories utilized while sleeping
B. Energy utilized to digest foods
C. Walking with her spouse in the evenings
D. Energy expended while tapping her foot

(D) Non-exercise activity thermogenesis (NEAT) is the energy expended for everything that does not include sleeping, eating, or dedicated physical exercise. NEAT includes many daily activities, ranging from yard work to fidgeting. These calories are generally not considered in the total energy expenditure formula. [Question 24]

References: Non-exercise activity thermogenesis (NEAT). Author: Levine, James. MD, PhD. Best Practice and Research Clinical Endocrinology and Metabolism. 2002 Dec; 16 (4):679-702.

178. (Content: II-C-3) A 43-year-old female presents with worsening acne over the past year. She has gained some weight, although she feels it has mostly accumulated in her abdomen. Which of the following tests is most appropriate at this time?

A. DHEA-S
B. MRI of the pituitary
C. Buccal salivary swab
D. Cosyntropin stimulation test

(C) Cushing's syndrome can be screened with a 24-hour urine free cortisol excretion, overnight 1 mg dexamethasone test, or a late-night buccal salivary swab. [Question 55]

Reference: Up to Date: "Establishing the diagnosis of Cushing's syndrome"

179. (Content: III-F-5b) A 39-year-old female presents to clinic with persistent symptoms of feeling flushed, lightheadedness, and some mild confusion. She underwent a sleeve gastrectomy one year prior but noted symptoms even before surgery. She is otherwise healthy, although she underwent a parathyroidectomy three months prior with recent electrolytes within normal limits. Which of the following is most likely associated with her findings?

A. **Elevated fasting c-peptide**
B. Female predominance of this disorder
C. Symptom improvement with increased protein intake
D. Normal fasting glucose with post-prandial hypoglycemia

(A) Multiple endocrine neoplasia type 1 presents with hyperparathyroidism, pituitary adenomas, and insulinomas. Insulinomas have elevated fasting c-peptide levels, with hypoglycemic episodes occurring irrespective of prior surgeries or food intake. [Question 167]

Reference: Rariy CM, Rometo D, Korytkowski M. Post-Gastric Bypass Hypoglycemia. Curr Diab Rep. 2016 Feb;16(2):19. doi: 10.1007/s11892-015-0711-5. PMID: 26868861.
Reference: Noninsulinoma pancreatogenous hypoglycemia syndrome on Up to Date

180. (Content: III-D-2) A 29-year-old male presents to an urgent care for COVID symptoms. He states that although he has no respiratory symptoms, his taste seems abnormal. He says it is particularly noticeable when drinking soda. His rapid COVID test is negative. Upon medication review, which of the following is most likely the culprit for his current symptoms?

A. Bupropion
B. Semaglutide
C. **Topiramate**
D. Phentermine

(C) Topiramate side effects include paresthesia, dysgeusia (abnormal taste), lightheadedness, and mental fogginess. [Question 105]

Reference: Phentermine/topiramate ER package insert

181. (Content: I-B-6) A 29-year-old female has been working vigorously over the past six months to increase her fitness level and decrease her weight before her upcoming wedding. After the wedding, she reduced her exercise routine to three times weekly and is frustrated she is starting to regain weight. Which of the following is likely to blame for her recent weight gain?

A. Adaptive thermogenesis
B. **Commitment amnesia**
C. Neurohurmonal influences
D. Increased muscle efficiency

(B) Commitment amnesia is one reason why patients may experience a weight plateau or experience weight gain. This concept refers to a lack of maintaining behavior, dietary, and physical activity levels required to lose the initial weight. [Question 40]

Reference: Obesity medicine association: Obesity Algorithm (2021)

182. (Content: III-F-3) A patient immediately after a Roux-en-Y surgery is difficult to extubate and eventually requires reintubation while still in the postanesthesia unit. A chest x-ray is normal, a complete blood count is normal, and a metabolic panel shows decreased bicarbonate. What is the most likely diagnosis?

A. Anastomotic leak
B. **Pulmonary embolism**
C. Obstructive sleep apnea
D. Pseudocholinesterase deficiency

(B) Failure to extubate should prompt an evaluation for a pulmonary embolism (PE) or an anastomotic leak. A pulmonary embolism presents with hypoxia and tachypnea (leading to respiratory alkalosis with compensatory metabolic acidosis). An anastomotic leak presents with leukocytosis and often a unilateral pleural effusion. [Question 211]

Reference: AACE/TOS/ASMBS/OMA/ASA 2019 Guidelines: CLINICAL PRACTICE GUIDELINES FOR THE PERIOPERATIVE NUTRITION, METABOLIC, AND NONSURGICAL SUPPORT OF PATIENTS UNDERGOING BARIATRIC PROCEDURES – 2019 UPDATE. Recommendation 47

183. (Content: I-C-1) Statistics are being evaluated to determine how income and education levels affect rates of obesity in adults. Which of the following would be expected to have the highest rates of obesity?

    A. Well-educated females
    B. Men living in poverty
    C. Men in the middle class
    D. Females in the middle class

(C) With women, increased obesity was seen in those with <u>more</u> poverty and <u>less</u> education. In men, more obesity is seen in <u>middle-class</u> incomes and those with <u>moderate</u> education (completed some college). [Question 31]

Reference: Ogden CL, Fakhouri TH, Carroll MD, et al. Prevalence of Obesity Among Adults, by Household Income and Education — United States, 2011–2014. MMWR Morb Mortal Wkly Rep 2017;66:1369–1373. DOI: **Reference:** NCHS, National Health and Nutrition Examination Survey, 2017–2018. https://www.cdc.gov/nchs/data/factsheets/factsheet_nhanes.htm

184. (Content: IV-B-1) Which of the following should be available in all physician's offices that treat patients with obesity?

    A. Exam tables that can accommodate 300 lbs
    B. Open scales available in public areas
    C. Chairs without side rails
    D. Sheets to cover the patients instead of gowns

(C) An office that is treating patients with obesity should have obesity-sensitive reading materials available in the waiting room, Furniture to accommodate > 300 lbs, wide chairs with handrails or standard chairs without side rails, exam tables with capacity up to 600 lbs, blood pressure cuffs and gowns in large and extra-large sizes, and scales that weigh up to 350 lbs- 700 lbs (calibrated monthly and located in a private area). Also, all staff should be trained in appropriate first-person language, free of bias, stigma, shaming, or embarrassment. [Question 224]

Reference: Toward Sensitive Treatment of Obese Patients; Syed M. Ahmed, MD, MPH, DrPH, Jeanne Parr Lemkau, PhD, and Sandra Lee Birt

185. (Content: I-A-3) Which pediatric condition is associated with enlarged organs and hepatoblastoma?

   A. Cohen syndrome
   B. Alstrom syndrome
   C. Beckwith-Wiedemann syndrome
   D. Prader-Willi syndrome

(C) Beckwith-Wiedemann syndrome is a fetal overgrowth syndrome that commonly presents with enlarged organs (hepatomegaly, splenomegaly, nephromegaly, and macroglossia) and predisposes the patient to tumor growth (i.e., hepatoblastoma). [Question 38]

Reference: Up to Date: "Beckwith-Wiedemann Syndrome"
Reference: Obesity medicine association: Pediatric Obesity Algorithm (2020-2022)

186. (Content: II-B-4) A metabolic and bariatric surgery center is evaluating a 44-year-old female. During the initial consult, she admits to eating until uncomfortably full and feeling guilty afterward. Although she states some of the guilt has caused her to seek bariatric surgery options, she denies any excessive exercise or dietary changes. What other item is she most likely to admit to?

   A. Hiding her eating behaviors
   B. Waking up in the night to eat
   C. Consuming most of her calories at night
   D. Induced vomiting after meals

(A) Binge eating disorder is a compulsive eating disorder characterized by marked distress about eating large amounts of food in a discrete amount of time with a sense of lack of control over eating during these episodes. It is associated with eating more rapidly than usual, until uncomfortably full, when not physically hungry, and hiding eating behaviors due to embarrassment. They feel disgusted, depressed, or guilty after episodes. [Question 46]

Reference: DSM-5: Diagnostic and Statistical Manual of Mental Disorders, Fifth Edition

187. (Content: III-D-2 and 9) A child has received a diagnosis of proopiomelanocortin deficiency. A melanocortin 4 receptor agonist will be initiated. Which other condition is this medication indicated?

    A. Leptin receptor deficiency
    B. Prader-Willi syndrome
    C. Class III pediatric obesity
    D. Alstrom syndrome

(A) Setmelanotide (Imcivree®) is a melanocortin 4 (MC4) receptor agonist approved for chronic weight management in those with genetically confirmed pathogenic proopiomelanocortin (POMC), proprotein convertase subtilisin/kexin type 1 (PCSK1) genes or leptin receptor (LEPR) deficiency. As of 2022, it is also approved for Bardet-Biedl syndrome. [Question 184]

Reference: Setmelanotide package inserts.
Reference: Ramos-Molina B, Martin MG, Lindberg I. PCSK1 Variants and Human Obesity. Prog Mol Biol Transl Sci. 2016;140:47-74. doi:10.1016/bs.pmbts.2015.12.001

188. (Content: II-D-2) What is the relationship between fat-free mass and lean body mass?

    A. Lean body mass and fat-free mass are within 15-20% of each other
    B. Lean body mass includes fat in the bone marrow and central nervous system
    C. Fat-free mass excludes nonessential fat but includes essential fat
    D. These terms are theoretical and not able to be detected on imaging

(B) Lean body mass is the total body mass (including muscles, internal organs, water, bones, ligaments, and tendons) minus nonessential or storage adipose tissue. It differs from fat-free mass because lean body mass includes <u>essential</u> fat in the bone marrow, central nervous system, and internal organs. Fat-free mass does not include <u>any</u> body fat. [Question 69]

Reference: Obesity medicine association: Obesity Algorithm (2021)

189. (Content: III-F-4) Immediately before bariatric surgery, the patient should do which of the following?

A. Take oral nonsteroidal anti-inflammatories
B. Perform deep breathing exercises
C. Start pharmacologic deep venous thrombosis prophylaxis
D. Be administered approximately 2 liters of lactated ringers

(B) Preoperative enhanced recovery after bariatric surgery (ERABS) clinical pathways should be implemented in all patients undergoing bariatric surgery to improve postoperative outcomes. Preoperative recommendations include deep breathing exercises, CPAP, incentive spirometry, leg exercises, H_2 blocker/PPI, carbohydrate loading, and pre-anesthesia medication. [Question 111]

Reference: AACE/TOS/ASMBS/OMA/ASA 2019 Guidelines: CLINICAL PRACTICE GUIDELINES FOR THE PERIOPERATIVE NUTRITION, METABOLIC, AND NONSURGICAL SUPPORT OF PATIENTS UNDERGOING BARIATRIC PROCEDURES – 2019 UPDATE. Recommendation 34, 35, 36, 40. Table 8.

190. (Content: III-B-1) A patient eats six servings of fruit per day. How many total calories does this add to his daily caloric intake?

A. 180 calories
B. 240 calories
C. 360 calories
D. 420 calories

(C) The idea of an exchange diet is to group foods according to their nutritional value. A list of foods that constitute a serving is available and useful for those who desire to substitute a food choice that may be higher in carbohydrates and calories for lower ones. Serving sizes likely will appear on boards to some extent, so having a basic understanding of how many calories and carbohydrates are in 1 serving of common food groups is essential. One serving of fruit is 60 kcal and 15 grams of carbohydrates. [Question 198]

Reference: Gray A, Threlkeld RJ. Nutritional Recommendations for Individuals with Diabetes. [Updated 2019 Oct 13]. In: Feingold KR, Anawalt B, Boyce A, et al., editors. Endotext [Internet]. South Dartmouth (MA): MDText.com, Inc.; 2000-. Available from: https://www.ncbi.nlm.nih.gov/books/NBK279012/

191. (Content: III-D-2) Which of the following patients who have failed lifestyle modifications meet the criteria for anti-obesity medications?

A. A patient with a BMI of 26 kg/m² who has a strong family history of obesity
B. A patient with a BMI of 28 kg/m² who has polycystic ovarian syndrome
C. A patient with a BMI of 29 kg/m² on pitavastatin
D. A patient with a BMI of 30 kg/m² who is a bodybuilder

(C) Pharmacotherapy is indicated in those with a BMI ≥ 30 kg/m² or ≥ 27 kg/m² with comorbidities. For example, a patient with dyslipidemia (on a statin) with a BMI ≥ 27 kg/m² meets the criteria. Importantly, a BMI of 30 kg/m² in a weigh-lifter may be exaggerated, and a waist circumference would better reflect his health risks. [Question 137]

Reference: 2013 AHA/ACC/TOS Guideline for the Management of Overweight and Obesity in Adults. A Report of the American College of Cardiology/American Heart Association Task Force on Practice Guidelines and The Obesity Society. Box 11-12.

192. (Content: III-B-4) A 26-year-old female presents to the dietician for an initial consult for weight management. She has a history of obstructive sleep apnea and recurrent abdominal intertrigo. She inquires about the most effective dietary plan. What is the best response?

A. Adherence to a dietary plan long-term is required to be successful
B. The Mediterranean diet is anti-inflammatory and would help with the intertrigo
C. Strict low carbohydrates would be preferred to help with initial rapid weight loss
D. Calorie restriction to 1500 kcal/day provides a consistent calorie deficit

(A) Although several diet plans are available, each with its benefits, a dietary plan that provides a caloric deficit and is sustainable long-term will provide the best results and health benefits. Patient preference must be taken into account. [Question 141]

Reference: AACE/ACE Guidelines: AMERICAN ASSOCIATION OF CLINICAL ENDOCRINOLOGISTS AND AMERICAN COLLEGE OF ENDOCRINOLOGY COMPREHENSIVE CLINICAL PRACTICE GUIDELINES FOR MEDICAL CARE OF PATIENTS WITH OBESITY (2016): Recommendation 47, 65-66.

193. (Content: III-D-3) A patient undergoing weight management with naltrexone/bupropion ER admits to relapsing with intravenous heroin. Her urine drug screen is positive for heroin and hydrocodone. She admits her last dose of heroin was last night, and she took hydrocodone this morning. Which of the following recommendation should be provided?

A. Stop your naltrexone/bupropion ER immediately
B. Change to naltrexone monotherapy, as it can be used to treat opioid use disorder
C. Decrease opioid use while discontinuing the anti-obesity medication
D. Change to bupropion ER monotherapy for continued weight benefits

(C) Naltrexone competes for opioid receptors and thus should not be used if concurrently taking opiates. The concern with naltrexone with current opioids is that the effect of the opiate is blunted; thus, patients take higher doses to experience the same efficacy. If naltrexone is discontinued while still on high doses of opiates, the patient is at high risk for overdose (as there are now more opioid receptors available to be activated). Although this medication should be stopped in this clinical vignette, it is vital to alert the patient to reduce their concurrent opioid (ideally discontinue it) due to the increased receptor activation after naltrexone is stopped. [Question 181]

Reference: Naltrexone/bupropion ER package insert

194. (Content: III-D-2) At what minimum glomerular filtration rate are all FDA-approved long-term weight loss medications approved without restriction in dosing?

A. 15 mL/min
B. 30 mL/min
C. 45 mL/min
D. 60 mL/min

(D) All FDA-approved weight-loss medications are permissible in those with a GFR >50 mL/min. [Question 108]

Reference: AACE/ACE Guidelines: AMERICAN ASSOCIATION OF CLINICAL ENDOCRINOLOGISTS AND AMERICAN COLLEGE OF ENDOCRINOLOGY COMPREHENSIVE CLINICAL PRACTICE GUIDELINES FOR MEDICAL CARE OF PATIENTS WITH OBESITY (2016): Recommendation 83-85

195. (Content: III-G-4) A patient presents to her family practitioner for general health counseling. Which of the following would be consistent with tertiary prevention?

- A. Education on the prevention of obesity
- B. Initiate lifestyle interventions to decrease weight
- C. Start pharmacotherapy to prevent weight-related complications
- **D. Initiate semaglutide to improve diabetes control**

(D) Tertiary prevention refers to appropriately treating a disease to eliminate or mitigate complications of an already diagnosed disease. Generally, tertiary prevention requires some form of intervention (surgery or medication) in addition to lifestyle changes. [Question 98]

Reference: AACE/ACE Guidelines: AMERICAN ASSOCIATION OF CLINICAL ENDOCRINOLOGISTS AND AMERICAN COLLEGE OF ENDOCRINOLOGY COMPREHENSIVE CLINICAL PRACTICE GUIDELINES FOR MEDICAL CARE OF PATIENTS WITH OBESITY (2016): Recommendation 2

196. (Content: III-G-3) A patient who successfully underwent bariatric surgery has been losing weight steadily. Which of the following should be recommended to this patient?

- A. Continue your current dietary and physical activity plan until you are at your goal weight
- **B. Intensify your exercise regimen as you continue to lose weight**
- C. Adjust caloric intake by 50 calories/day until consistently losing weight
- D. Continue a liquid diet until at target weight, then introduce solids

(B) Patients who lose weight are often disheartened when they eventually plateau and experience some weight gain if their treatment regimen isn't adjusted. This should be discussed early in treatment to prevent frustration, with pre-emptive plans to adapt and intensify their regimen accordingly. Physical activity, in particular, helps avoid weight re-gain. [Question 122]

Reference: The National Weight Control Registry Brown Medical School/The Miriam Hospital. Weight Control & Diabetes Research Center

197. (Content: III-D-1) A 41-year-old patient, who was started on liraglutide two months prior for weight loss, is admitted to the emergency department with severe right-sided flank pain and hematuria. A renal stone passes the following day spontaneously. What is the most likely mechanism liraglutide contributed to her presentation?

A. Rapid weight loss
B. Volume contraction
C. Increased oxalate absorption
D. Reduced calcium excretion

(B) Although GLP-1 receptor agonists, such as liraglutide, do not directly cause kidney stones, a relatively common side effect is gastrointestinal distress. Nausea, vomiting, and diarrhea may cause hypovolemia, increasing the risk of nephrolithiasis. [Question 152]

Reference: AACE/ACE Guidelines: AMERICAN ASSOCIATION OF CLINICAL ENDOCRINOLOGISTS AND AMERICAN COLLEGE OF ENDOCRINOLOGY COMPREHENSIVE CLINICAL PRACTICE GUIDELINES FOR MEDICAL CARE OF PATIENTS WITH OBESITY (2016). Recommendation 86 and 87.

198. (Content: III-H-3) What is the minimal Tanner stage required in an adolescent to meet metabolic and bariatric surgery criteria?

A. Tanner Stage 1
B. Tanner Stage 2
C. Tanner Stage 3
D. Tanner Stage 4

(A) Pubertal status or physical maturity (Tanner Stage or bone age) are no longer included in determining surgery candidacy. Therefore, a patient with a Tanner Stage 1 would be a candidate for surgery as long as they meet other surgical criteria. [Question 194]

Reference: Obesity medicine association: Pediatric Obesity Algorithm (2020-2022)
Reference: Pratt JSA, Browne A, Browne NT, et al. ASMBS pediatric metabolic and bariatric surgery guidelines, 2018. Surg Obes Relat Dis. 2018;14(7):882-901. doi:10.1016/j.soard.2018.03.019

199. (Content: IV-A-1) What term best describes when a victim becomes the target of unfavorable treatment?

A. Stigma
B. Prejudice
C. Harassment
D. Bias

(D) Bias is the action that occurs when emotions result from stigma (disgust, anger, blame, etc.), leading to prejudice or unfavorable treatment. [Question 217]

Reference: Puhl RM, Heuer CA. Obesity stigma: important considerations for public health. Am J Public Health. 2010;100(6):1019-1028. doi:10.2105/AJPH.2009.159491

200. (Content: IV-A-3) A 17-year-old female presents with migraines and excess weight. She is interested in starting topiramate, as her mother had improvements with this medication. The patient is sexually active, uses condoms occasionally, and refuses to use birth control regularly. The physician refuses to prescribe topiramate. What ethical principle is involved in this decision?

A. Justice
B. Nonmaleficence
C. Autonomy
D. Beneficence

*(B) Ethical principles include respecting the patient's decision to refuse or accept treatments based on their preferences (autonomy), doing what is best for the patient (beneficence), doing no harm (nonmaleficence), and treating and providing care fairly to all patients (justice). In this case, the risk of birth defects is too high compared to the benefit, falling under the principle of **nonmaleficence.** [Question 220]*

Reference: Pratt JSA, Browne A, Browne NT, et al. ASMBS pediatric metabolic and bariatric surgery guidelines, 2018. Surg Obes Relat Dis. 2018;14(7):882-901. doi:10.1016/j.soard.2018.03.019

201. (Content: III-F-1) A patient plans to undergo metabolic and bariatric surgery within the next three months. If found upon endoscopy, which of the following should a Roux-en-Y gastric bypass be recommended over a sleeve gastrectomy?

A. Intestinal metaplasia in the esophagus
B. Gastric food remnants, despite being NPO for 12 hours
C. Helical-shaped, gram-negative bacteria in the stomach
D. Visible scarring from a previous PEG tube

(A) Roux-en-Y gastric bypass is the bariatric surgery of choice for patients with moderate-severe gastroesophageal reflux symptoms, hiatal hernia, esophagitis, or Barrett's esophagus (intestinal metaplasia). [Question 216]

Reference: AACE/ACE Guidelines: AMERICAN ASSOCIATION OF CLINICAL ENDOCRINOLOGISTS AND AMERICAN COLLEGE OF ENDOCRINOLOGY COMPREHENSIVE CLINICAL PRACTICE GUIDELINES FOR MEDICAL CARE OF PATIENTS WITH OBESITY (2016): Recommendation 62.

202. (Content: II-C-3 and 5) A 7-year-old male is sent to an endocrinologist due to abnormal electrolytes, including hypocalcemia and hyperphosphatemia. He has round facies, a high body mass index, and shorter stature. Which of the following conditions is most associated with these findings?

A. Albright-Hereditary Osteodystrophy
B. Prader-Willi syndrome
C. Proopiomelanocortin gene mutation
D. Bardet-Biedl syndrome

(A) Albright-Hereditary Osteodystrophy is characterized by a shorter stature, round facies, shortened fourth and fifth metacarpals, intellectual disability, impaired olfaction, and pseudohypoparathyroidism. Pseudohypoparathyroidism is characterized by renal resistance to parathyroid hormone (PTH), leading to hypocalcemia, hyperphosphatemia, and elevated PTH levels. [Question 96]

Reference: Obesity medicine association: Obesity Algorithm (2021)

203. (Content: III-F-4) A patient presents for a metabolic surgery screening consultation with an obesity medicine specialist. She does have slight hirsutism and admits to irregular periods. She also has striae on her abdomen. She has not been in a structured weight program previously. Which of the following should be recommended at this time?

A. Minimum weight loss of 15 lbs (6.8 kg) before surgery
B. Testing for sex hormonal abnormalities
C. Overnight dexamethasone suppression test
D. Six months of a structured weight loss program

(B) Testing for sex hormone abnormalities (total/bioavailable testosterone, DHEA-S, and 4-androstenedione) can be done if there is a suspicion for polycystic ovarian syndrome such as virilization. Screening for Cushing syndrome should be conducted if there are <u>wide</u>-based (>1cm) purple striae with other findings suggestive of hypercortisolism. There is no evidence to support mandatory strict weight loss amounts or specific durations of weight loss programs preoperatively. [Question 178]

Reference: AACE/TOS/ASMBS/OMA/ASA 2019 Guidelines: CLINICAL PRACTICE GUIDELINES FOR THE PERIOPERATIVE NUTRITION, METABOLIC, AND NONSURGICAL SUPPORT OF PATIENTS UNDERGOING BARIATRIC PROCEDURES – 2019 UPDATE. Table 7. Recommendation 13, 26, 27, 30, 31

204. (Content: III-F-1 and 2) An endoscopically placed weight loss device that can remain in place for one year, and works by helping delay the gastric transit of food content, describes which of the following?

A. Aspiration device
B. Intragastric balloon
C. TransPyloric Shuttle
D. Sleeve gastroplasty

(C) The TransPyloric Shuttle (TPS®) is an endoscopically-placed weight loss device that was FDA approved in 2019, which uses a removable gastric bulb to affect the flow of food content through the stomach. [Question 175]

Reference: FDA- TransPyloric Shuttle/TransPyloric Shuttle Delivery Device - P180024

205. (Content: III-D-5) A male patient presents to his primary care physician complaining of excessive burping. Recently, he started supplements to help with weight loss. Which of the following supplements is most likely contributing to his presentation?

    A. Glucosinolates
    B. Green tea extract
    C. Raspberry ketones
    D. Chitosan

(C) A side effect of raspberry extract is significant burping, whereas chitosan causes indigestion, bloating, and constipation. Glucosinolates can cause goiters and hypothyroidism. [Question 200]

Reference: Obesity medicine association: Obesity Algorithm (2021)

206. (Content: III-D-3) The maximum dose of bupropion in the combination anti-obesity medication Naltrexone/bupropion ER (Contrave®) is between what values?

    A. 0-100 mg/day
    B. 100-200 mg/day
    C. 200-300 mg/day
    D. 300-400 mg/day

(D) The maximum dose of Naltrexone/bupropion ER (Contrave®) is 2 tablets twice daily, with each tablet consisting of 8 mg naltrexone/90 mg bupropion ER, for a total of 32 mg naltrexone and 360 mg bupropion ER daily. [Question 181]

Reference: Naltrexone/bupropion ER package insert

207. (Content: III-D-5) A patient is interested in starting semaglutide (Wegovy®). The maximum weekly dose, if tolerated, is between which of the following ranges?

A. 0.5 to 1 mg
B. 1 to 1.5 mg
C. 1.5 to 2 mg
D. 2 to 2.5 mg

(D) Semaglutide (Wegovy®) is a once-weekly GLP-1 receptor agonist injected subcutaneously. Patients should inject 0.25 mg subcutaneously weekly for one month and increase the dose to 0.5 mg, 1.0 mg, 1.7mg, and 2.4 mg weekly (maximum dose) at one-month intervals. [Question 124]

Reference: Semaglutide package insert.

208. (Content: III-G-7) Appropriate testosterone replacement in a male with hypogonadism is most likely to improve which of the following conditions?

A. Blood pressure
B. Lipid panel
C. Sleep apnea
D. Fertility

(B) Testosterone replacement is associated with weight loss, decreased waist circumference, reduced fertility, and improvements in glucose, HbA1c, and cholesterol. [Question 107]

Reference: AACE/ACE Guidelines: AMERICAN ASSOCIATION OF CLINICAL ENDOCRINOLOGISTS AND AMERICAN COLLEGE OF ENDOCRINOLOGY COMPREHENSIVE CLINICAL PRACTICE GUIDELINES FOR MEDICAL CARE OF PATIENTS WITH OBESITY (2016): Recommendation 54

209. (Content: I-B-4) A recently married male presents for discussion of increased weight gain. He states since moving in with his wife, he feels more fatigued and hungrier throughout the daytime. He goes to bed and wakes up at similar times compared to before marriage. He was tested for sleep apnea one year ago, which was negative. What other question may help to determine his increased appetite?

A. Have you had recent thyroid studies?
B. Does your wife have restless leg syndrome?
C. Do you take melatonin before bedtime?
D. Was the sleep study done in a sleep center or at home?

(B) Decreased sleep duration or reduced sleep quality strongly correlates with increased orexigenic hormones leading to increased appetite, hunger, and ultimately weight. Interruptions of sleep may occur from restless leg syndrome, obstructive sleep apnea, bed partner movements including animals, circadian misalignment, and sleep-maintenance insomnia. For this patient, if the timing correlates, his wife may have restless leg syndrome reducing his sleep quality. [Question 6]

Reference: Jean-Louis G, Williams NJ, Sarpong D, Pandey A, Youngstedt S, Zizi F, Ogedegbe G. Associations between inadequate sleep and obesity in the US adult population: analysis of the national health interview survey (1977-2009). BMC Public Health. 2014 Mar 29;14:290. doi: 10.1186/1471-2458-14-290. PMID: 24678583; PMCID: PMC3999886.

210. (Content: III-D-8) Which class of medications used for diabetes prevents the breakdown of the incretins glucagon-like peptide 1 and gastric inhibitory peptide, increasing pancreatic insulin synthesis and decreasing glucagon?

A. DDP-4 inhibitors
B. SGLT2- inhibitors
C. Metformin
D. Sulfonylureas

(A) Dipeptidyl Peptidase 4 (DPP-4) inhibitors prevent the breakdown of incretins glucagon-like peptide 1 and gastric inhibitory peptide, increasing pancreatic insulin synthesis and decreasing glucagon. [Question 114]

Reference: Sitagliptin package insert

211. (Content: IV-A-3) The principle of "doing what is best for the patient" falls under which ethical principle?

A. Justice
B. Nonmaleficence
C. Autonomy
D. Beneficence

(D) Ethical principles include respecting the patient's decision to refuse or accept treatments based on their preferences (autonomy), doing what is best for the patient (beneficence), doing no harm (nonmaleficence), and treating and providing care fairly to all patients (justice). [Question 220]

Reference: Pratt JSA, Browne A, Browne NT, et al. ASMBS pediatric metabolic and bariatric surgery guidelines, 2018. Surg Obes Relat Dis. 2018;14(7):882-901. doi:10.1016/j.soard.2018.03.019

212. (Content: III-C-1) "Perform 45 minutes of water walking at 2 miles per hour every Monday, Wednesday, and Friday before work. In addition, lift weights for 15 minutes on days that you do not swim." This statement describes which of the following?

A. A SMART goal
B. An exercise prescription
C. 'Arrange/Assist' component of the 5 A's of obesity management
D. Component of motivational interviewing

(B) An exercise prescription is a physical activity plan customized based on patients' preferences and abilities to provide specific activities to perform. The prescription components should include frequency, intensity, time, type, and enjoyment. [Question 155]

Reference: Physical Activity Guidelines for Americans: 2nd Edition: https://health.gov/sites/default/files/2019-09/Physical_Activity_Guidelines_2nd_edition.pdf

213. (Content: II-D-2) A male presents to an obesity medicine clinic as he was told that he was considered to have obesity based on his percentage of fat. Which of the following is the minimum percentage of body fat to meet this criterion in this patient?

A. 23%
B. 28%
C. 32%
D. 38%

(B) Percent body fat can assist in diagnosing patients with obesity, defined as ≥ 25% percent body fat in males and ≥ 32% in females. [Question 50]

Reference: Obesity Medicine Association: Obesity Algorithm (2021)

214. (Content: III-G-3) A 15-year-old female who underwent a sleeve gastrectomy nine months prior is returning due to increasing weight over the prior two months. Although she no longer runs outside due to the cold winter, she has maintained 300 mins/week of moderate physical activity at the gym. She denies other stressors. Which of the following should be recommended at this time?

A. Strict documentation of calorie intake
B. Increasing physical activity by 20%
C. Surgery re-evaluation for potential anatomic etiology
D. Laboratory assessment

(A) Insufficient weight loss or weight regain after bariatric surgery can be from many etiologies, with the most common etiology being behavioral mediated. This includes lack of dietary control (i.e., snacking), nonadherence with calorie-restriction recommendations, lack of exercise, or increased psychosocial stressors. Especially over the holidays (winter months), calories may increase inadvertently. [Question 190]

Reference: Up to Date: "Bariatric surgery: Postoperative and long-term management of the uncomplicated patient"

215. (Content: I-A-3) A 6-year-old male patient presents to the pediatrician for recurrent shoulder dislocations. His joints are hypermobile. He is minimally interactive and does not make eye contact but has an open-mouth expression. His vision is poor. He has thickened hair and eyebrows. This condition is characterized by what genetic abnormality?

A. Autosomal dominant
B. Autosomal recessive
C. X-linked recessive
D. X-linked dominant

(B) Cohen syndrome is an autosomal recessive genetic cause of obesity. It is associated with small head size, narrow hands and feet, joint hypermobility, "open mouth" expression, a low white blood cell count, retinal dystrophy, and thick hair and eyebrows. [Questions 23 and 38]

Reference: Up To Date: "Genetic contribution and pathophysiology of obesity."
Reference: Obesity medicine association: Pediatric Obesity Algorithm (2020-2022)

216. (Content: II-A-3) A 26-year-old male, not on any medications, has a diagnosis of metabolic syndrome according to the National Cholesterol Education Program (NCEP) Adult Treatment Panel III (ATP III). Which of the following characteristics is likely to be present in this patient?

A. Triglycerides of 140 mg/dL (reference range < 150 mg/dL)
B. HbA1c of 6.1% (reference range < 5.7%)
C. Total cholesterol of 210 mg/dL (reference range <200 mg/dL)
D. Blood pressure of 128/80 mmHg

(B) Diagnostic criteria for metabolic syndrome are based on the presence of at least 3 of the following: abdominal obesity, hypertriglyceridemia, low serum high-density lipoprotein (HDL) cholesterol, elevated blood pressure, and increased fasting plasma glucose (corresponds to HbA1c ≥ 5.7%). [Question 60]

Reference: Up to Date: "Metabolic syndrome (insulin resistance syndrome or syndrome X)"

217. (Content: I-A-4) An 11-year-old female is diagnosed with new-onset hypertension and prediabetes. Upon further workup, an adrenal adenoma secreting excess cortisol is discovered. Which of the following growth chart characteristics is likely seen in this patient?

    A. Proportional weight and height increases
    B. Increased height compared to weight
    C. Normal growth charts
    D. Increased weight compared to height

(D) In contrast to children with excess weight due to increased caloric intake, those with endocrinopathies such as hypercortisolism or thyroid disorders will significantly increase weight compared to height. [Question 21]

Reference: Obesity medicine association: Pediatric Obesity Algorithm (2020-2022)

218. (Content: I-B-8) Exogenous leptin is injected into a test subject. This hormone is found to stimulate which of the following pathways?

    A. Cocaine and amphetamine-regulated transcript
    B. Neuropeptide Y
    C. Agouti-related peptide
    D. Y1 and Y5 receptors

(A) Leptin inhibits neuropeptide Y/agouti-related peptide first-order neurons of the orexigenic pathway and stimulates the proopiomelanocortin/cocaine and amphetamine-regulated transcript first-order neurons within the anorexigenic pathway. [Question 8]

Reference: Varela L, Horvath TL. Leptin and insulin pathways in POMC and AgRP neurons that modulate energy balance and glucose homeostasis. EMBO Rep. 2012;13(12):1079-1086. doi:10.1038/embor.2012.174

219. (Content: II-D-3a) A patient is asked a series of questions about the likelihood of falling asleep during certain activities throughout the day. These questions are screening for a condition directly associated with which of the following parameters?

   A. Elevated FVC/FEV$_1$ ratio
   B. Increased respiratory disturbance index
   C. Elevated daytime carbon dioxide
   D. Prolonged QRS interval

(B) The Epworth Sleepiness Scale is a clinical pretest probability scoring system used for obstructive sleep apnea (OSA) screening. It includes a series of questions pertaining to the likelihood of them falling asleep during certain activities throughout the day. OSA is associated with an increased respiratory disturbance index and apnea-hypopnea index. [Questions 52 and 88]

Reference: Up To Date: "Clinical manifestations and diagnosis of OSA in adults"
Reference: AACE/ACE Guidelines: AMERICAN ASSOCIATION OF CLINICAL ENDOCRINOLOGISTS AND AMERICAN COLLEGE OF ENDOCRINOLOGY COMPREHENSIVE CLINICAL PRACTICE GUIDELINES FOR MEDICAL CARE OF PATIENTS WITH OBESITY (2016). Recommendation 21.

220. (Content: III-E) A patient starts taking a daily pill that she states is advertised to help stimulate healthy intestinal bacterial growth, which promotes a microbiome conducive to weight loss. Which of the following does this describe?

   A. Dietary fiber
   B. Oligosaccharides
   C. Probiotics
   D. Stool softener

(B) Prebiotics are indigestible oligosaccharides that may stimulate healthy intestinal bacterial growth, promoting a microbiome conducive to weight loss. Probiotics are 'healthy bacteria' such as lactobacilli. [Question 131]

Reference: Obesity medicine association: Obesity Algorithm (2021)

221. (Content: III-F-5a) Which of the following statements is true regarding the use of warfarin in patients who have undergone bariatric surgery and developed postoperative venous thromboembolism (VTE)?

A. Warfarin is preferred because it can be monitored closely
B. Warfarin should never be used after a gastric bypass
C. In the setting of an acute DVT, bridge warfarin with enoxaparin
D. Avoid using warfarin initially, but it is still an option

(D) Perioperative VTE treatment recommendations include using parenteral anticoagulation in the early/subacute phase after bariatric surgery (<4 weeks), with a transition to direct oral anticoagulation or vitamin K antagonists being considered after at least four weeks of parenteral therapy. Closely monitor levels of oral anticoagulation to ensure absorption and adequate bioavailability. [Question 112]

Reference: Martin KA, Beyer-Westendorf J, Davidson BL, Huisman MV, Sandset PM, Moll S. Use of direct oral anticoagulants in patients with obesity for treatment and prevention of venous thromboembolism: Updated communication from the ISTH SSC Subcommittee on Control of Anticoagulation. J Thromb Haemost. 2021 Aug;19(8):1874-1882. doi: 10.1111/jth.15358. Epub 2021 Jul 14. PMID: 34259389.

222. (Content: II-A-3) A 32-year-old male presents to the clinic to inquire about injectable weight loss medications. In particular, he is interested in one that is also used in diabetes. Which of the following may be a contraindication of this medication?

A. Pituitary adenoma
B. Calcitonin elevation
C. History of volvulus
D. Glaucoma

(B) Contraindications to GLP-1 receptor agonists (GLP-1 RA) include prior hypersensitivity to medication class, history or family history of medullary thyroid carcinoma (calcitonin is a tumor marker for this malignancy), patients with multiple endocrine neoplasia type 2, and pregnancy. Relative contraindications include severe gastroparesis and increased risk of pancreatitis (although meta-analysis has not shown an increased risk of pancreatitis or pancreatic cancer with GLP-1 RA use). [Question 73]

Reference: Liraglutide package insert

223. (Content: III-D-2) Patients with which of the following comorbidities should cellulose and citric acid be avoided?

A. **Plummer Vinson syndrome**
B. Gastrointestinal reflux disease
C. Celiac disease
D. Irritable bowel syndrome

(A) Patients with active esophageal abnormalities (such as rings or webs in Plummer Vinson syndrome), gastrointestinal strictures, or other complications from gastrointestinal anatomical abnormalities that may inhibit transit or motility should avoid volume-occupying treatments such as cellulose and citric acid hydrogel (brand name Plenity®). [Question 179]

Reference: Cellulose and Citric Acid Hydrogel package insert

224. (Content: IV-E-2) An administrator is trying to determine the extra cost burden for employees that have the disease of obesity. He has categorized costs into indirect and direct. In this scenario, an example of indirect costs would include which of the following?

A. **Absenteeism**
B. Physician visits
C. Prescription drug use
D. Hospitalizations

(A) Indirect costs related to excess weight are associated with decreased productivity in the workplace. This includes absenteeism (lost production to the employee not being at work), presenteeism (decreased productivity while at work), premature disability, and mortality. [Question 222]

Reference: Obesity and Presenteeism: The Impact of Body Mass Index on Workplace Productivity. Journal of Occupational and Environmental Medicine: January 2008 - Volume 50 - Issue 1 - p 39-45;
Reference: Annual medical spending attributable to obesity: payer-and service-specific estimates. Health Aff (Millwood). 2009 Sep-Oct;28(5):w822-31. doi: 10.1377/hlthaff.28.5.w822. Finkelstein EA1, Trogdon JG, Cohen JW, Dietz W

225. (Content: III-A-1 and 2) A female is presenting for her three-month follow-up appointment. Over the past two years, she has successfully lost 45 lbs (20.4 kg). As the holidays are coming, she is fearful as she knows this is her most challenging time regarding excess eating due to the number of family events scheduled. Which of the following questions is most appropriate?

A. Given your weight loss, don't you feel like you deserve to reward yourself?
B. What is your goal weight after the holidays?
C. **Are there any other family members going through a similar weight loss journey?**
D. What could you eat before the event to curb your appetite?

(C) Motivational interviewing and cognitive-behavioral therapy (CBT) lead to higher patient engagement and ownership, decreasing resistance/barriers and improving overall outcomes. CBT focuses on changing behaviors through cognitive restructuring to reinforce good behaviors and extinguish undesirable ones. One of the components of cognitive-behavioral therapy includes enlisting social support. [Questions 110 and 127]

Reference: Dalle Grave R, Centis E, Marzocchi R, El Ghoch M, Marchesini G. Major factors for facilitating change in behavioral strategies to reduce obesity. Psychol Res Behav Manag. 2013;6:101-110. Published 2013 Oct 3. doi:10.2147/PRBM.S40460
Reference: Obesity Medicine Association: Obesity Algorithm (2021)

226. (Content: I-A-3) A research study recruits 1,000 individuals with the disease of obesity. What is the highest prevalence gene most likely seen in this population?

A. LEPR
B. **FTO**
C. MC4R
D. POMC

(B) FTO variant gene expression is the most common genetic finding in patients with obesity in the general population. It is related to a higher BMI and waist circumference. [Question 2]

Reference: Up To Date: "Genetic contribution and pathophysiology of obesity"

227. (Content: I-D-4) The United States Department of Agriculture provides what acceptable macronutrient distribution range for fat intake?

A. 5-15%
B. 15-25%
C. 25-35%
D. 35-40%

(C) The USDA provides acceptable macronutrient distribution ranges, including protein intake of 10-35%, carbohydrate intake of 45-65%, and fat intake of 25-35%. [Question 44]

Reference: Dietary Reference Intakes for Energy, Carbohydrate, Fiber, Fat, Fatty Acids, Cholesterol, Protein, and Amino Acids (2005)

228. (Content: III-H-3) A 14-year-old female, with the agreement of her parents, has decided to pursue a sleeve gastrectomy due to her persistently elevated body mass index, pre-diabetes, and obstructive sleep apnea. Which of the following would be a contraindication to surgery?

A. Heroin use 2 months ago
B. A BMI in the 125% of the 95th percentile
C. Tanner Stage 2
D. Alcohol use within the past month

(A) Contraindications to bariatric surgery are similar in adolescents and adults. They include ongoing substance abuse history (within 1 year), medically correctable causes of obesity, current or planned pregnancy within 12-18 months of surgery, any condition (medical, psychiatric, psychosocial, or cognitive) that prevents adherence to the post-operative regimen. [Question 194]

Reference: Obesity medicine association: Pediatric Obesity Algorithm (2020-2022)
Reference: Pratt JSA, Browne A, Browne NT, et al. ASMBS pediatric metabolic and bariatric surgery guidelines, 2018. Surg Obes Relat Dis. 2018;14(7):882-901. doi:10.1016/j.soard.2018.03.019

229. (Content II-C-1) A patient has a one-month follow-up visit for new-onset hypertension. He states he feels well and denies any new complaints. A review of records shows a body mass index (BMI) increase of 3 kg/m^2 over the past month without an increase in waist circumference. Persistent trace edema is present. Which of the following conditions likely led to his increased BMI?

A. Nephrotic syndrome
B. Vertebral compression fracture
C. Seasonal clothing changes
D. Increased dietary intake

(A) Any condition that increases excess water through third spacing (i.e., cirrhosis, nephrotic syndrome, heart failure) tends to overestimate BMI but not increase adiposity-related risk factors usually associated with an increased BMI. [Question 64]

Reference: Obesity medicine association: Obesity Algorithm (2021)
Reference: Up to Date: "Obesity in adults: Prevalence, screening, and evaluation"

230. (Content: III-B-1) A 66-year-old female has read about a new diet plan that restricts fruits but allows increased protein intake. She feels this would be a good fit, as she has a barbeque business. Which of the following is this dietary plan most similar to?

A. Dietary approach to stop hypertension (DASH)
B. Paleo diet
C. Carbohydrate restricted diet
D. Mediterranean diet

(C) In a carbohydrate-restrictive diet (< 45% calories from carbs), fruits, dairy, carbohydrates, and starchy vegetables are restricted. [Question 97]

Reference: Obesity medicine association: Obesity Algorithm (2021)

231. (Content: III-E) What is one of the potentially negative effects of oxyntomodulin?

A. Blockade of GLP-1 receptors
B. Increased risk of gallstones
C. Glucagon agonist
D. Hypoglycemic effects

(C) Oxyntomodulin has agonist effects on glucagon-like peptide 1 (GLP-1) and glucagon receptors. Although the GLP-1 effects are desirable, glucagon counters insulin secretion and increases circulating glucose levels. Fortunately, the more pronounced GLP-1 effects counterbalance this deleterious effect. [Question 172]

Reference: Pocai A. Action and therapeutic potential of oxyntomodulin. Mol Metab. 2013;3(3):241-251. Published 2013 Dec 14. doi:10.1016/j.molmet.2013.12.001
Reference: Obesity Medical Association: Obesity Algorithm 2021

232. (Content: II-B-3) A 24-year-old male is found deep within the woods. He states he wanted to go on a 3-month camping trip in which he secluded himself from the world and lived "off the land." He previously had minimal experience camping and stated he mostly consumed fish and occasional rabbits. He avoided berries or plants as he was unsure which were safe to eat. Which of the following is likely to be seen on physical examination?

A. Night blindness
B. Perifollicular hemorrhage
C. Anasarca
D. Koilonychia

(B) Scurvy, due to severe vitamin C deficiency, has symptoms that include anemia, perifollicular microhemorrhages, weakness/fatigue, poor wound healing, petechia, ecchymosis, bleeding gums, and dry skin. [Question 80]

Reference: Léger D. Scurvy: reemergence of nutritional deficiencies. Can Fam Physician. 2008;54(10):1403–1406.

233. (Content: III-B-1) The recommended daily caloric intake for females to obtain an energy deficit of at least 500 kcal/day is closest to which of the following?

    A. 900 kcal/day
    B. 1100 kcal/day
    C. 1300 kcal/day
    D. 1600 kcal/day

(C) An energy deficit of ≥ 500 kcal/day is recommended for weight loss and may be achieved with a daily caloric intake for males of 1500-1800 kcal/d and females of 1200-1500 kcal/d. [Question 208]

Reference: 2013 AHA/ACC/TOS Guideline for the Management of Overweight and Obesity in Adults. A Report of the American College of Cardiology/American Heart Association Task Force on Practice Guidelines and The Obesity Society. Box 9.

234. (Content: III-F-5b) A patient status-post Roux-en-Y gastric bypass complains of lightheadedness and flushing after meals. In terms of timing, how could post-gastric bypass hypoglycemia (PGBH) and early dumping syndrome (DS) be differentiated?

    A. DS occurs 1-4 hours after meals
    B. PGBH is generally seen > 1 year after surgery
    C. Symptoms of dumping syndrome last for > 30 minutes
    D. PGBH symptoms can persist for > 4 hours

(B) Post-gastric bypass hypoglycemia is thought to be due to a persistent increase in incretins (GLP-1 and GIP) post-operatively, leading to hyperfunctioning/hypertrophied β-islet cells. This, along with improved insulin sensitivity with weight loss, may lead to symptoms. It presents with delayed post-prandial hypoglycemia (1-4 hours postoperatively), most often occurring >1 year after surgery. Early dumping syndrome is usually seen within the first postoperative year and occurs within 15-30 minutes of a meal. [Question 167]

Reference: Rariy CM, Rometo D, Korytkowski M. Post-Gastric Bypass Hypoglycemia. Curr Diab Rep. 2016 Feb;16(2):19. doi: 10.1007/s11892-015-0711-5. PMID: 26868861.
Reference: Noninsulinoma pancreatogenous hypoglycemia syndrome on Up to Date

235. (Content: III-A-1) A patient presents for dietary follow-up. Although he has changed his eating habits to include more fruits, vegetables, and avoidance of soda, he has not appreciated much improvement in his weight. He is frustrated and states, "I will never lose weight. These changes were a waste of time." The dietician states, "You have already shown a lot of initiative in your lifestyle modifications. Let's see how we can channel that to other areas like physical activity." What motivational interview principle was displayed?

A. Empathy
B. Avoiding arguments
C. Resolving ambivalence
D. Developing discrepancy

(B) Avoiding arguments is a motivational interview principle that includes "Rolling with resistance" through reflection, shifting the focus, reframing, and siding with the negative. [Question 161]

Reference: Obesity medicine association: Obesity Algorithm (2021)

236. (Content: I-B-1 and I-A-1 and 3) A 27-year-old female with a BMI of 29 kg/m^2 presents for pre-conception counseling. Her smartwatch has been calculating approximately 5 hours of sleep nightly. What findings would be expected to increase if she improved her nightly sleep duration?

A. Ghrelin
B. Neuropeptide Y
C. Proopiomelanocortin
D. Melanin-concentrating hormone

(C) Sleep deprivation and reduced sleep quality are associated with decreased leptin levels, leading to increased appetite and reduced energy expenditure. This stimulates the orexigenic hormones. In contrast, if sleep quality is improved, anorexigenic hormones, such as proopiomelanocortin, will increase as leptin levels improve. [Questions 19 and 30]

Reference: Mignot, Emmanuel, et al. Stanford.edu/med-sleep-1208.html, Dec 2004
Reference: Varela L, Horvath TL. Leptin and insulin pathways in POMC and AgRP neurons that modulate energy balance and glucose homeostasis. EMBO Rep. 2012;13(12):1079-1086. doi:10.1038/embor.2012.174

237. (Content: I-B-6) A pathologist uses a special dye within the pancreas to identify prominent areas of hormone secretion. The stain for amylin would be seen within which cells?

   A. Alpha cells
   B. Beta cells
   C. Delta cells
   D. Gamma cells

(B) Amylin is secreted by the pancreas' beta islet cells and is co-secreted with insulin. In type 2 diabetes, insulin and amylin levels are increased, although they are less effective (i.e., resistance). [Question 17]

Reference: Erin E. Kershaw, Jeffrey S. Flier, Adipose Tissue as an Endocrine Organ, The Journal of Clinical Endocrinology & Metabolism, Volume 89, Issue 6, 1 June 2004, Pages 2548–2556, https://doi.org/10.1210/jc.2004-0395

238. (Content: III-F-2) A surgeon has collaborated with an anesthesiologist for pre-operative evaluation for patients planning to undergo metabolic and bariatric surgery. The assessment will be completed one week before the surgery date. Which of the following patients should have surgery delayed or canceled due to an elevated perioperative risk?

   A. A patient over the age of 65 years old with sleep apnea
   B. A patient who quit smoking cigarettes 3 months ago
   C. A patient with factor 5 Leiden deficiency on apixaban
   D. A female who stopped oral contraceptives 1 week ago

(D) Estrogen products should be stopped for one cycle of oral contraceptives (premenopausal) or three weeks of hormone replacement therapy (postmenopausal) to reduce the risk of post-procedure thrombosis. [Question 140]

Reference: AACE/TOS/ASMBS/OMA/ASA 2019 Guidelines: CLINICAL PRACTICE GUIDELINES FOR THE PERIOPERATIVE NUTRITION, METABOLIC, AND NONSURGICAL SUPPORT OF PATIENTS UNDERGOING BARIATRIC PROCEDURES – 2019 UPDATE. Recommendation 2, 17, 18, 23, 33

239. (Content: II-B-2) A 45-year-old male with a BMI of 62 kg/m² presents for a follow-up visit regarding his weight. Since his last visit, he has increased his water walking to 1 hour per day, four days during the week, and has maintained a 1600 kcal/day caloric intake. What would be the best advice to provide at this time?

    A. Increase water walking to 5 days per week
    B. Restrict calories an additional 400 kcal/day
    C. Lift weights on weekends
    D. Walk on the treadmill on days when not water walking

(C) The minimum physical activity goal should be ≥ 150 min/week of moderate-intensity exercise, performed during 3-5 sessions per week. In addition, resistance training should be prescribed to those undergoing weight-loss therapy to promote fat loss while preserving fat-free mass (goal 2-3x weekly). [Question 89]

Reference: AACE/ACE Guidelines: AMERICAN ASSOCIATION OF CLINICAL ENDOCRINOLOGISTS AND AMERICAN COLLEGE OF ENDOCRINOLOGY COMPREHENSIVE CLINICAL PRACTICE GUIDELINES FOR MEDICAL CARE OF PATIENTS WITH OBESITY (2016): Recommendation 67- 70

240. (Content: I-B-5) A patient is undergoing testing to determine their total energy expenditure (TEE). The value of energy expenditure from physical activity is estimated to be which approximate percentage of TEE?

    A. 10%
    B. 25%
    C. 40%
    D. 60%

(B) Total energy expenditure is made up of the following components: resting energy expenditure (60-75%), thermic effect of meals (10%), and energy expenditure from physical activity (15-30%). [Question 4]

Reference: Obesity medicine association: Obesity Algorithm (2021)

241. (Content: II-D-2) A bodybuilder undergoes a program to improve strength and endurance. Measurements are taken throughout the 12-week course to see the progression. In particular, his percent body fat is measured. What formula best describes this measurement?

A. Total mass – fat mass
B. **Fat mass/(total body mass – bone mass)**
C. Total mass – fat mass – bone mineral content
D. Fat mass + lean mass + bone mass

(B) The calculation to determine percent body fat = fat mass/(total body mass – bone mass). Fat-free mass is calculated by taking total mass minus fat mass. Total body mass is the total sum of fat mass, lean mass, and bone mass. [Question 69]

Reference: Obesity medicine association: Obesity Algorithm (2021)

242. (Content: I-D-1) During a lifestyle improvement lecture, a dietician recommends that a daily intake of 400 international units of vitamin D would be sufficient to meet the requirements of nearly all healthy, non-pregnant female patients. This amount of vitamin D meets the criteria for which of the following?

A. Daily value
B. **Recommended dietary allowance**
C. Estimated average requirement
D. Adequate intake

(B) Recommended dietary allowance (RDA) is the average daily dietary intake of a nutrient that is sufficient to meet the requirements of nearly all healthy persons within a particular population (age, gender, pregnancy, elderly, etc.). [Question 13]

Reference: National Agricultural Library: U.S. Department of Agriculture

243. (Content: III-H-4) A mother asks her family practitioner how to assist her 11-year-old daughter in maintaining a healthy weight. During the COVID pandemic, the daughter reduced her physical activity and increased her caloric intake. This has led to increased weight. Which of the following is the best advice?

A. Encourage her to jog for 1 hour daily in the evening or morning
B. Allow the patient to eat more frequent smaller meals
C. **Exchange one restaurant meal for a home-cooked family meal**
D. Encourage her to reduce her time in front of her bedroom television

(C) Integrating the family into a healthier initiative will prevent the child from feeling singled out, especially younger females. This could include family walks and changing dietary plans. Avoid allowing children to have televisions in bedrooms, and allow the child to assist in physical activity plans with activities they enjoy. [Question 151]

Reference: Expert Committee Recommendations Regarding the Prevention, Assessment, and Treatment of Child and Adolescent Overweight and Obesity: Summary Report and APPENDIX. Sarah E. Barlow and the Expert Committee; Pediatrics December 2007, 120 (Supplement 4) S164-S192; DOI: https://doi.org/10.1542/peds.2007-2329C.

244. (Content: I-D-2) A 49-year-old patient with long-standing diabetes, controlled on metformin for the past seven years, presents for follow-up after being told she has "low blood counts" during a life-insurance screening exam. Given her medical history, what vitamin should be checked?

A. Iron
B. Folate
C. **Cyanocobalamin**
D. Copper

(C) Metformin interferes with B_{12} absorption in the ileum. Prolonged use is associated with B_{12} deficiency. B_{12} deficiency can cause pancytopenia, macrocytosis, and subacute combined degeneration. [Question 27]

Reference: Up to Date: "Causes and pathophysiology of vitamin B_{12} and folate deficiencies"
Reference: Up to Date: "Bariatric surgery: Postoperative nutritional management"

245. (Content: II-D-1) A weight management clinic is discussing options to determine metabolic rate. Which statement is most accurate regarding the relationship between resting metabolic rate (RMR) and basal metabolic rate (BMR)?

    A. BMR is easier to obtain in an office setting
    B. RMR requires an individual to be fasting
    C. Total energy expenditure is based on BMR only
    D. BMR and RMR are both increased with increased weight

(D) Basal metabolic rate (BMR) is similar to resting metabolic rate (RMR) but requires the individual to be fasting, resting, and supine in a thermoneutral environment. Both BMR and RMR are increased in the setting of increased body weight. [Question 86]

Reference: **Reference:** Obesity medicine association: Obesity Algorithm (2021)

246. (Content: III-A-1) A 19-year-old has recently started eating healthy and initiated a physical activity plan at his university this past month. He has never been in a program like this but is enjoying it, and he wants to be able to participate in intermural sports in the upcoming season. Which of the following would be important to help in his current goals at this stage?

    A. Build awareness and discuss risks and benefits
    B. Set goals and develop an action plan
    C. Reward and encourage small changes
    D. Discuss lapse and relapse coaching

(C) The stages of change include pre-contemplation, contemplation, preparation, action, and maintenance. The action phase refers to the initiation of change (approx. 6 months), and the intervention includes cognitive behavioral therapy, in particular rewarding and encouraging small changes. [Question 116]

Reference: **Reference:** Obesity Medicine Association: Obesity Algorithm (2021)

247. (Content: III-F-5c) A patient presents with peripheral edema, neuropathy, and a new S3 on physical examination. Upon further review, the patient has been consuming a severely calorie-deficient diet to lose weight over an extended period. Based on symptoms, what deficiency is likely present?

A. Mineral
B. Fat-soluble vitamin
C. Total protein
D. **Water-soluble vitamin**

(D) Dry beriberi presents with symmetric peripheral polyneuropathy (sensory and motor), mostly affecting the distal extremities. It results from thiamine (B_1) deficiency, a water-soluble vitamin. [Question 104]

Reference: Up to Date: "Overview of water-soluble vitamins"

248. (Content: III-F-4) The enhanced recovery after bariatric surgery (ERABS) recommendations include

A. **administering intra-operative regional blocks**
B. increasing tidal volume to maximally tolerated
C. delaying post-operative oral intake until bowel function returns
D. providing preoperative blood transfusion to improve hemodynamics

(A) Preoperative enhanced recovery after bariatric surgery (ERABS) clinical pathways should be implemented in all patients undergoing bariatric surgery to improve postoperative outcomes. Intraoperatively, this includes opioid-sparing multi-modal analgesia, pulmonary recruitment maneuvers and protective ventilation strategies, silent bleeding detection, avoiding excess fluid administration (goal-directed fluid management), anti-emetic prophylaxis, and regional blocks. [Question 111]

Reference: AACE/TOS/ASMBS/OMA/ASA 2019 Guidelines: CLINICAL PRACTICE GUIDELINES FOR THE PERIOPERATIVE NUTRITION, METABOLIC, AND NONSURGICAL SUPPORT OF PATIENTS UNDERGOING BARIATRIC PROCEDURES – 2019 UPDATE. Recommendation 34, 35, 36, 40. Table 8.

249. (Content: I-B-3) A 47-year-old male presents to his cardiologist for an annual evaluation. The prior year, he underwent a successful right coronary artery stent for stable coronary artery disease. Which anthropometric measurements would be the best predictor of future mortality?

A. **Waist circumference**
B. Body mass index
C. Resting metabolic rate
D. Skin fold calipers

(A) Patients with increased waist circumference had higher associated 5-year mortality throughout all BMI ranges. [Question 36]

Reference: Combining Body Mass Index With Measures of Central Obesity in the Assessment of Mortality in Subjects With Coronary Disease; Thais Coutinho, Kashish Goel, Daniel Corrêa de Sá, Rickey E. Carter, David O. Hodge, Charlotte Kragelund, Alka M. Kanaya, Marianne Zeller, Jong Seon Park, Lars Kober, Christian Torp-Pedersen, Yves Cottin, Luc Lorgis, Sang-Hee Lee, Young-Jo Kim, Randal Thomas, Véronique L. Roger, Virend K. Somers, Francisco Lopez-Jimenez; J Am Coll Cardiol. 2013 Feb, 61 (5) 553-560.

250. (Content: III-F-1) The trend of Roux-en-Y gastric bypass (RYGB) over the past ten years is best described by which of the following sentences?

A. The numbers of RYGB declined initially, followed by a steady incline.
B. RYGB makes up approximately half of the bariatric surgeries.
C. **The percentage of RYGB is now similar to the percentage of bariatric revisions.**
D. The number of RYGB has continued to increase in the pediatric patient population.

(C) Although the total number of bariatric surgeries has increased, it is mainly from the increased popularity of the sleeve gastrectomy (61% of surgeries). RYGB has continued to decline, making up 17% of the total bariatric surgeries, similar to bariatric revisions (15.4% in 2018, which continues to increase). [Question 136]

Reference: https://asmbs.org/resources/estimate-of-bariatric-surgery-numbers

251. (Content: II-D-2) Which patient characteristic would have a relatively higher lean body mass?

A. Male gender
B. Older individual
C. Sedentary individual
D. Patient with cachexia

(A) Lean body mass is less in females, those who are sedentary, and decreases with age. As most lean body mass is made up of muscle (40%), an increase in lean body mass is often a marker of increased muscle mass. Therefore, if you think of patients with increased muscle mass, you can more easily identify which characteristics of patients would have increased lean body mass. Higher lean body mass is associated with increased health, whereas higher fat mass is associated with increased health risks. Males have increased lean body mass when compared to females. [Question 69]

Reference: Obesity medicine association: Obesity Algorithm (2021)

252. (Content: III-D-3) A patient presents to the emergency department with persistent fatigue, loss of appetite, and anasarca. Labs reveal a high anion gap metabolic acidosis and renal failure. Which of the following medications most likely led to the acid-base disorder?

A. Metformin
B. Topiramate
C. Phentermine
D. Bupropion

(A) Metformin may cause lactic acidosis, especially in the setting of renal failure. Lactic acidosis causes a high anion gap metabolic acidosis, whereas topiramate causes a hyperchloremic metabolic acidosis (non-anion gap metabolic acidosis). [Question 203]

Reference: Metformin and topiramate package inserts

253. (Content: III-B-2 and III-G-2) A very motivated patient presents to the clinic in January after making a New Year's Resolution for weight loss. He wants to be aggressive with his approach and has researched a very low-calorie diet (VLCD). What is an appropriate statement about this approach?

    A. It has been shown to have greater long-term weight effects
    B. A VLCD tends to be more cost-effective
    C. Complication risks are eliminated if monitored monthly
    D. Patients on this diet intake significant amounts of protein

(D) A very low-calorie diet (VLCD) is any diet under 800 kcal/day which requires close monitoring to reduce the risk of complications. The typical diet consists of a predominance of protein (suppresses hunger). There is little evidence to support that a VLCD is superior to a low-calorie diet (800 -1500 kcal/day), and the two approaches have no increased long-term weight benefits. Despite close monitoring, several complications such as electrolyte abnormalities, gout flares, and cholelithiasis may occur. Interestingly, the cost is generally increased in VLCD due to commonly utilizing strict packaged meal replacements and more frequent follow-up visits. [Question 201]

Reference: Up to Date: "Obesity in adults: Dietary therapy"
Reference: Moreno B, Bellido D, Sajoux I, Goday A, Saavedra D, Crujeiras AB, Casanueva FF. Comparison of a very low-calorie-ketogenic diet with a standard low-calorie diet in the treatment of obesity. Endocrine. 2014 Dec;47(3):793-805. doi: 10.1007/s12020-014-0192-3. Epub 2014 Mar 4. PMID: 24584583.

254. (Content: III-D-3) A 44-year-old female recently started on semaglutide for diabetes and concurrent weight loss. Which of the following parameters will likely increase as a result of starting this therapy?

    A. HDL cholesterol
    B. Triglycerides
    C. Hemoglobin A1c
    D. Diastolic blood pressure

(A) Regarding studies on anti-obesity medications, GLP-1 receptor agonists, bupropion SR/ naltrexone, and phentermine/topiramate ER all increased HDL and lowered LDL, triglycerides, and hemoglobin A1c. In addition, all improved systolic blood pressure except bupropion SR/naltrexone. [Question 162]

Reference: Vorsanger MH, Subramanyam P, Weintraub HS, Lamm SH, Underberg JA, Gianos E, Goldberg IJ, Schwartzbard AZ. Cardiovascular Effects of the New Weight Loss Agents. J Am Coll Cardiol. 2016 Aug 23;68(8):849-59. doi: 10.1016/j.jacc.2016.06.007. PMID: 27539178.

255. (Content: I-B-4) A 39-year-old female presents with painful bumps that begin to develop over the thighs and abdomen. On examination, multiple discrete subcutaneous nodules are palpable, ranging in size from 3-6 mm. What is the most likely etiology of this finding?

A. **Dercum's disease**
B. Lipedema
C. Lymphedema
D. Lipodystrophy

(A) Adiposis dolorosa, also known as Dercum's disease, occurs most commonly in women 30-50 years old affected by obesity. It is characterized by painful lipomas that can occur anywhere on the body but are most commonly present on the torso or proximal extremities. [Question 11]

Reference: https://rarediseases.org/rare-diseases/dercums-disease/

256. (Content: II-B-3) A 45-year-old male with class II obesity presents to the emergency department in cardiac arrest. Family members state he went on an extreme diet, only drinking water for the past three weeks. He had lost a significant amount of weight but became weak and irritable, per the family. Today he decided to break his fast by ordering a pizza. Shortly after his meal, he became unconscious, and an ambulance was called. What deficiency most likely lead to his current condition?

A. **Phosphate**
B. Thiamine
C. Calcium
D. Potassium

(A) Refeeding syndrome is a life-threatening condition in severely malnourished people. This occurs in the setting of prolonged malnutrition leading to depleted phosphate storage. If provided unrestricted nutrition, especially high in carbohydrates, insulin release causes phosphate to shift intracellularly. Because phosphate is used for energy in the form of ATP, muscle weakness (including cardiac and diaphragm) and fatal arrhythmias can occur. [Question 80]

Reference: Up to Date: "Hypophosphatemia: Causes of hypophosphatemia"

257. (Content: III-B-1) A 49-year-old female with a history of type II diabetes presents to her primary care clinician to discuss her recent lab work. She is currently on metformin and her most recent hemoglobin A1c was 9.1% (reference range < 5.7%). She is planning to start a ketogenic diet to help with diabetes control but is also open to starting a new medication. Which of the following classes of medications should be avoided at this time?

A. GLP-1 receptor agonist
B. DPP4 inhibitor
C. SGLT-2 inhibitor
D. Thiazolidinedione

(C) Extreme caution should be used if a patient is starting a ketogenic diet and is currently taking an SGLT-2 inhibitor due to the risk of ketoacidosis. Ideally, this class of medication would be discontinued. Insulin should also be decreased, with hypoglycemic education provided and close monitoring recommended. [Question 97]

Reference: Obesity medicine association: Obesity Algorithm (2021)

258. (Content: I-B-5) In calculating the resting energy expenditure, which of the following components plays the most prominent role in the Mifflin St. Jeor equation equation?

A. Age
B. Gender
C. Weight
D. Height

(C) Although all of the above components are considered in both the Harris-Benedict and Mifflin St. Jeor equations, weight plays the most influential role. In the Mifflin St. Jeor equation, it is multiplied by a factor of 10. The equation is: Resting energy expenditure = (10 x Weight) + (6.25 x Height) - (5 x Age) + Gender factor. For the gender factor, for females, subtract 161, and for males, add 5. You do not need to memorize these calculations for ABOM. However, knowing which components are in the equation and which plays the most significant role (weight) is essential. In addition, know that the Mifflin-St. Jeor equation is more accurate in those with obesity. [Question 4]

Reference: Mifflin MD, St Jeor ST, Hill LA, et al. A new predictive equation for resting energy expenditure in healthy individuals. Am J Clin Nutr. 1990 Feb;51(2):241-7. PubMed ID: 2305711

259. (Content: II-C-5) A young child was recently diagnosed with Angelman syndrome. What is the genetic etiology of this condition?

A. Autosomal recessive
B. **Maternal imprinting error**
C. Paternal deletion of 15q13
D. Trisomy

(B) Angelman syndrome is caused by a genetic abnormality of chromosome 15 called the ubiquitin protein ligase E3A (UBE3A), which is normally inherited from the mother (maternal imprinting) whereas the paternal gene is normally silenced. However, if the mother's gene is missing or defective, this causes Angelman syndrome. A similar paternal deletion of a gene in this same location causes Prader-Willi syndrome. [Question 72]

Reference: Up To Date "Microdeletion syndromes (chromosomes 12 to 22)"
Reference: https://www.mayoclinic.org/diseases-conditions/angelman-syndrome/symptoms-causes/syc-20355621

260. (Content: III-F-5a) A 29-year-old female presents to her obstetrician for her 20-week fetal ultrasound evaluation. She became pregnant two months after a Roux-en-Y gastric bypass and takes bariatric vitamins sporadically. During the exam, a fetal abnormality is noted on the midline of the spine. Intake of which of the following vitamins would have prevented this complication?

A. **Folate**
B. Cyanocobalamin
C. Thiamine
D. Copper

(A) Females should wait 12-18 months after bariatric surgery to become pregnant due to the increased risk of vitamin deficiencies. In particular, folate deficiency can lead to neural tube defects in the fetus. [Question 65]

Reference: Up to Date: "Overview of water-soluble vitamins"

261. (Content: I-B-7) A study is being conducted to determine the differences in hormone levels in men versus women at equivalent body mass index values. It will likely be found that compared to women, men have

A. higher levels of adiponectin
B. **lower levels of leptin**
C. equivalent sex hormone binding globulin levels
D. decreased lean body mass

(B) With obesity, leptin levels increase in both men and women. However, at equivalent body mass index levels, men have lower leptin and adiponectin levels. [Question 29]

Reference: Kennedy A, Gettys TW, Watson P, Wallace P, Ganaway E, Pan Q, Garvey WT. The metabolic significance of leptin in humans: gender-based differences in relationship to adiposity, insulin sensitivity, and energy expenditure. J Clin Endocrinol Metab. 1997 Apr;82(4):1293-300. doi: 10.1210/jcem.82.4.3859. PMID: 9100610.

262. (Content: III-C-1) A 20-year-old female presents to discuss exercise recommendations. She is planning to perform 300 minutes of moderate-intensity exercise weekly. She would like to target a specific heart rate to determine her level of physical intensity. What is the recommended heart rate to target for moderate-intensity exercise?

A. 100 BPM (50% of max predicted heart rate)
B. 120 BPM (60% of max predicted heart rate)
C. **140 BPM (70% of max predicted heart rate)**
D. 160 BPM (80% of max predicted heart rate)

(C) Moderate-intensity exercise is described as being 3-6 METS. At this level of intensity, a conversation takes effort (you can talk but not sing), an example being a brisk walk. The heart rate target for this intensity is between 64-76% of the maximum predicted heart rate. Maximum predicted heart rate is estimated by 220 - age. So for this patient, maximum predicted heart rate is 220 – 20 = 200, with a target heart rate for modeterate intensity exercise between 120 (200 x 0.64) and 152 (200 x 0.76) beats per minute. [Question 117]

Reference: CDC: Target Heart Rate and Estimated Maximum Heart Rate.
https://www.cdc.gov/physicalactivity/basics/measuring/heartrate.htm

263. (Content: III-D-8) Which of the following medications used for diabetes is considered weight-neutral?

A. Metformin
B. Sitagliptin
C. Exenatide
D. Glipizide

(B) Dipeptidyl Peptidase 4 (DPP-4) inhibitors like sitagliptin are considered weight neutral, while metformin and exenatide (GLP-1 receptor agonist) are considered weight negative. Glipizide, a sulfonylurea is obesogenic. [Question 114]

Reference: Sitagliptin package insert

264. (Content: I-A-3) What inheritance pattern is Wilson-Turner syndrome?

A. Autosomal dominant
B. Autosomal recessive
C. X-Linked
D. Trisomy

(C) Wilson-Turner syndrome and Fragile X syndrome display X-linked inheritance patterns. Wilson-Turner syndrome is a rare disease characterized by predominantly truncal obesity, short stature, gynecomastia, hypogonadism, and dysmorphic facial features, including a broad nasal tip, mandibular hypoplasia, deep sunken eyes, and thickened eyebrows. [Question 38]

Reference: National Center for Advancing Translational Sciences:
https://rarediseases.info.nih.gov/diseases/5579/wilson-turner-syndrome

265. (Content: I-A-2) A study utilizing a functional MRI is being conducted. Images of food are displayed to the research participant while they are in an MRI. The researcher can visualize activated areas within the brain in real time. One particular image activates the amygdala. Which of the following qualities about the food image likely caused this activation?

A. A memory associated with the image
B. A prior food addiction
C. Ghrelin stimulation of NPY/AgRP
D. **A successful advertisement**

(D) The amygdala activates in response to food cues (advertisements, visual, etc.) and is part of the hedonic, not the homeostatic pathway (i.e., NPY/AgRP). The limbic system is mediated by cravings, rewards, and addiction, while food memories activate the hippocampus. [Question 37]

Reference: Farr OM, Li CR, Mantzoros CS. Central nervous system regulation of eating: Insights from human brain imaging. Metabolism. 2016 May;65(5):699-713. doi: 10.1016/j.metabol.2016.02.002. Epub 2016 Feb 6. PMID: 27085777; PMCID: PMC4834455.

266. (Content: II-A-3) A study comparing the relative risk of mortality between those with a normal BMI and those with a BMI $\geq$ 40 kg/m^2 is most likely to discover that females with higher BMIs have a greater relative risk of which cancer?

A. Colon
B. **Endometrial**
C. Pancreatic
D. Breast

(B) Females with a BMI $\geq$ 40 kg/m^2 are 7 times more likely to develop endometrial cancer than those with a lower BMI. The relative risks of other malignancies related to excess weight include esophageal (4.8x), gastric, liver and kidney (2x), pancreatic (1.5x), breast (1.4x), and colorectal (1.3x). [Question 183]

Reference: Obesity and Cancer: National Cancer Institute: https://www.cancer.gov/about-cancer/causes-prevention/risk/obesity/obesity-fact-sheet

267. (Content: II-D-1) Which of the following patients is most likely to have a higher VO₂ max?

A. **A 23-year-old male who swims 30 minutes daily**
B. A 65-year-old female who walks 2 miles daily
C. A 50-year-old male with a body fat percentage of 36%
D. A 33-year-old male with Down syndrome

(A) The volume of oxygen consumed (VO₂) is a marker of oxygen utilization, with higher levels indicating increased efficiency. In general, levels decrease with age, with approximately a 30% decrease at age 65 compared to age 20. Athletes have higher VO₂ levels as decreased body fat percentage increases levels. Males generally have higher VO₂ levels, when compared to females. Therefore, of the options, a 23-year-old male who swims 30 minutes daily would have higher levels as he is younger, male, and physically active. [Question 62]

Reference: Lundby C, Montero D, Joyner M. Biology of VO2 max: looking under the physiology lamp. Acta Physiol (Oxf). 2017 Jun;220(2):218-228. doi: 10.1111/apha.12827. Epub 2016 Nov 25. PMID: 27888580.

268. (Content: III-G-7) A 68-year-old male with class II obesity underwent a heart catheterization after having a stress test showing reversible myocardial ischemia. He is started on aspirin and clopidogrel. The cardiologist asks you to start a beta-blocker. Which of the following is the most appropriate medication to start?

A. **Carvedilol**
B. Metoprolol succinate
C. Atenolol
D. Metoprolol tartrate

(A) Some beta-blockers such as atenolol, propranolol, and metoprolol increase adipose tissue, leading to increased weight. If patients require beta blockers, carvedilol is the most weight-neutral option. [Question 165]

Reference: Obesity medicine association: Obesity Algorithm (2021)

269. (Content: III-H-2) A 12-year-old male is being treated for a genetic cause of obesity. The medication has worked well, but the child admits to having spontaneous erections that have become bothersome. Which of the following medications is he most likely taking?

A. Metreleptin
B. Setmelanotide
C. Semaglutide
D. Tirzepatide

(B) Significant adverse reactions associated with setmelanotide include new or worsening depression or suicidal ideation, increased sexual arousal (labial hypersensitivity and priapism), and skin hyperpigmentation. Sexual arousal is due to increased sympathetic activation of the melanocortin 4 receptor. [Question 184]

Reference: Setmelanotide package inserts.

270. (Content: III-G-5) A 56-year-old female underwent a sleeve gastrectomy two years prior and has lost nearly 100 lbs (45.5 kg) since surgery. She feels tired, wakes up with night sweats, and continues to lose weight. She has a decreased appetite but denies stomach pains. She continues to lose weight and is now in the underweight category. All vitamin and laboratory work is normal. What is the most likely etiology of her symptoms?

A. Menopause
B. Underlying malignancy
C. Dumping syndrome
D. Depression

(B) Excessive weight loss and malnourishment after bariatric surgery should be evaluated. Some causes include eating disorders such as bulimia or anorexia nervosa, underlying malignancy (associated with increased fatigue, night sweats, and potentially localizing symptoms, etc.), small intestinal bowel overgrowth (symptoms would include bloating, nausea, early satiety, abdominal discomfort, and diarrhea), anastomotic stricture (symptoms include localized abdominal pain, food aversion, and possibly dysphagia), and depression or other psychiatric conditions. [Question 57]

Reference: Akusoba I, Birriel TJ, El Chaar M. Management of Excessive Weight Loss Following Laparoscopic Roux-en-Y Gastric Bypass: Clinical Algorithm and Surgical Techniques. Obes Surg. 2016 Jan;26(1):5-11. doi: 10.1007/s11695-015-1775-7. PMID: 26105983.

271. (Content: I-D-4) A patient intakes 10 grams of carbohydrates. How many kcal did they consume?

A. 20 kcal
B. 40 kcal
C. 70 kcal
D. 90 kcal

(B) Both carbohydrates and proteins have 4 kcal/gm, compared to fat having 9 kcal/gm and alcohol having 7 kcal/gm. Given this patient consumed 10 grams of carbohydrates, they consumed 40 kcal (4 kcal/gm x 10 gm). [Question 44]

Reference: Dietary Reference Intakes for Energy, Carbohydrate, Fiber, Fat, Fatty Acids, Cholesterol, Protein, and Amino Acids (2005)

272. (Content: I-A-5) A 21-year-old female patient is discussing weight during pre-conception counseling. She has a strong family history of obesity, although she and her husband have normal body mass indexes. Which of the following could contribute to the risk of obesity in her children later in life?

A. Exclusively breastfeeding for the first six months
B. Physical abuse in the household
C. Education within a private school setting
D. Vaginal delivery causing a perineal laceration

(B) Adverse childhood events (ACE) can contribute to excess weight gain during childhood and even into adulthood. The highest contributing factors include the death of a parent, witnessing or experiencing violence or abuse, and financial constraints. The higher number of ACE, the more likely affected individuals will develop obesity due to its cumulative effect. [Question 5]

Reference: Elsenburg LK, van Wijk KJE, Liefbroer AC, Smidt N. Accumulation of adverse childhood events and overweight in children: A systematic review and meta-analysis. Obesity (Silver Spring). 2017 May;25(5):820-832. doi: 10.1002/oby.21797. Epub 2017 Apr 3. PMID: 28371524.

273. (Content: III-G-7) A 39-year-old male presents to the clinic for headaches. He has a history of hypogonadism treated with intramuscular testosterone and obstructive sleep apnea treated with continuous positive airway pressure. He underwent a sleeve gastrectomy the year prior and lost 62 lbs (28.1 kg). Labs reveal a hemoglobin level of 19.3 g/dL (reference range: 13.5–17.5 g/dL) with a low erythropoietin level. What is the most important next step?

A. Obtain a renal ultrasound
B. Repeat levels in 1 month
C. Reduce the testosterone dose
D. Repeat a sleep study

(C) In this patient who has lost significant weight, the dose of testosterone likely needs to be reduced, as testosterone levels increase with weight loss. Erythropoietin would be expected to be increased in the setting of renal cell carcinoma or untreated sleep apnea and suppressed in testosterone-induced polycythemia, a secondary cause. [Question 107]

Reference: Kelly DM, Jones TH. Testosterone and obesity. Obes Rev. 2015 Jul;16(7):581-606. doi: 10.1111/obr.12282. Epub 2015 May 15. PMID: 25982085.

274. (Content: III-A-1) A physician is seeing a patient in the bariatric clinic. The patient states that "weight loss is as simple as calories in and calories out." The physician resists the desire to correct him but instead tries to understand where the patient is coming from. This motivational technique is best described by which of the following models?

A. OARS
B. RULE
C. FRAMES
D. PACE

*(B) **RULE** is an acronym focused on the motivation interview principles, and stands for **R**esist the righting reflex, **U**nderstand your patient's motivation, **L**isten to your patient, and **E**mpower your patient. [Question 110]*

Reference: Obesity Medicine Association: Obesity Algorithm (2021)

275. (Content: III-F-3) A 21-year-old male begins complaining of significant abdominal pain 48 hours after undergoing a successful Roux-en-Y gastric bypass. A barium study reveals an anastomotic leak at the gastrojejunostomy anastomosis site. Which of the following is likely present in this patient?

    A. Dilated loops of bowel
    B. Unilateral pleural effusion
    C. Decreased perfusion in the mesenteric arteries
    D. Abnormality on EKG

(B) Anastomotic leaks usually occur within the first few days of surgery. It often presents with a reactive pleural effusion and leukocytosis. [Question 120]

Reference: Obesity medicine association: Obesity Algorithm (2021)

276. (Content: III-D-4) A patient is started on 3 mg daily of oral semaglutide. The patient returns for follow-up lab work; the hemoglobin A1c is the same as it was before beginning semaglutide, three months prior. What is the reason for this lack of improvement?

    A. The starting dose has no glucose control
    B. This medication is only used for weight-loss
    C. This patient is a non-responder to therapy
    D. The hemoglobin A1c was checked too soon

(A) The oral form of semaglutide (Rybelsus®) is taken daily, with the initial dose (3 mg daily for 30 days) being used only to improve gastrointestinal tolerance but provides no significant glucose control. Therefore, up-titration to 7 mg or 14 mg is necessary for glucose improvement. [Question 209]

Reference: Semaglutide package inserts.

277. (Content: III-F-5a) A 16-year-old male is seen in the hospital on post-operative day one from a sleeve gastrectomy. In addition to abdominal pain, he complains of abdominal bloating, weakness, and dizziness while standing. Orthostatic vital signs are positive. What is the most appropriate test to order at this time?

- A. D-dimer
- **B. Hemoglobin**
- C. Chest x-ray
- D. Basic metabolic panel

(B) Intraluminal bleeding (presents as hematemesis or hematochezia) or intra-abdominal bleeding (increased abdominal fullness) is a short-term complication of any surgery, including metabolic and bariatric surgery. If suspected, obtain a hemoglobin level, and notify the surgeon. [Question 120]

Reference: Obesity medicine association: Obesity Algorithm (2021)

278. (Content: III-D-5) A 39-year-old female with a past medical history of obesity class II and familial hypercholesteremia presents for follow-up after increasing her semaglutide level to the maximum dose for weight loss. Which of the following side effects is she most likely to be experiencing?

- **A. Constipation**
- B. Cold intolerance
- C. Palpitations
- D. Hirsutism

(A) GLP-1 receptor agonists commonly cause gastrointestinal side effects due to decreased intestinal motility. This may cause nausea, vomiting, abdominal discomfort, and dose-dependent constipation. Ensuring adequate hydration, as well as utilizing laxatives, may be necessary. [Question 124]

Reference: Semaglutide package insert

279. (Content: III-D-2 and 9) Which of the following conditions is setmelanotide approved for?

    A. Albright hereditary osteodystrophy
    B. Angelman syndrome
    C. Congenital leptin deficiency
    D. Bardet-Biedl

(D) Setmelanotide is approved for patients ≥ 6 years old with pathogenic POMC, PCSK1, or LEPR genetic defects, in addition to a recent indication for Bardet-Biedl syndrome (2022). [Question 184]

Reference: Setmelanotide package inserts.

280. (Content: III-B-4) A patient presents to discuss different dietary options. She is particularly interested in initiating a low-fat diet. Which of the following is the most important piece of information to provide?

    A. Target a reduction in your polyunsaturated intake
    B. Replace saturated fats with refined carbohydrates
    C. A lower-fat diet increases total cholesterol but decreases LDL
    D. Replace saturated fats with whole grains

(D) Replacing saturated fats with whole grain carbohydrates reduces coronary heart disease (CHD) by 9%, whereas exchanging them with refined carbohydrates increases CHD slightly, and is not recommended. Reducing fat intake helps lower LDL and total cholesterol; substituting polyunsaturated fats in place of saturated fats has been shown to reduce CHD by 30%, similar to statin therapy. [Question 148]

Reference: Dietary Fats and Cardiovascular Disease: A Presidential Advisory from the American Heart Association. Circulation 2017;Jun 15:
Reference: Up to Date: "Dietary fat"

281. (Content: II-D-2) A study is being performed correlating increased percent body fat in those with metabolic syndrome. A direct correlation is found among different ethnic groups. Comparatively, which population would have higher rates of metabolic syndrome?

A. African American men
B. Hispanic women
C. Caucasian women
D. Asian men

(B) Caucasian males tend to have higher rates of percent body fat and metabolic syndrome, with the prevalence lower in African American males. Similarly, Hispanic females generally had higher rates than Caucasian females. [Question 50]

Reference: Obesity Medicine Association: Obesity Algorithm (2021)
Reference: Ford ES, Li C, Zhao G. Prevalence and correlates of metabolic syndrome based on a harmonious definition among adults in the US. J Diabetes. 2010 Sep;2(3):180-93. doi: 10.1111/j.1753-0407.2010.00078.x. PMID: 20923483.

282. (Content: III-G-7) A 46-year-old with recurrent migraines is presenting to discuss treatment options. She has tried topiramate but did not tolerate the side effects at the dose required to prevent migraines effectively. She is adamant about not wanting to start a medication that causes weight gain. Which of the following would be contraindicated, given her wishes?

A. Erenumab
B. Botox injections
C. Valproic acid
D. Zonisamide

(C) All options above can be used to prevent migraines and are considered weight-neutral or even weight-negative (zonisamide) except for valproic acid. If possible, this medication should be avoided in those who are at risk for developing weight gain. [Question 189]

Reference: Obesity medicine association: Obesity Algorithm (2021)

283. (Content: III-G-7) An abdominal waist circumference is being performed on a patient prior to a referral to a renal transplant program. How should this measurement be completed to yield the most accurate results?

- A. The measuring tape should be taut and compress the skin
- **B. The measurement should be done at the level of the iliac crest**
- C. The measurement should be done right after normal inspiration
- D. The measuring tape should be at the level of the umbilicus

(B) For the most accurate results, abdominal waist circumference should be obtained at the level of the iliac crest. The measuring tape should be parallel to the floor and snug without compressing the skin. The measurement taken at the end of normal expiration is the most precise. [Question 49]

Reference: Obesity medicine association: Obesity Algorithm (2021)

284. (Content: III-F-3) A 39-year-old female presents as an acute visit to the bariatric surgeon's office. The patient had undergone a Roux-en-Y gastric bypass three weeks prior. For the past five days she has had epigastric abdominal pain and progressively worsening nausea and vomiting. Vital signs are unremarkable. A barium study and upper endoscopy were unremarkable. Laboratory work, including a complete blood count, was normal. What is the most likely etiology of her symptoms?

- A. Anastomotic leak
- **B. Mesenteric thrombosis**
- C. Marginal ulcer
- D. Intraabdominal abscess

(B) Mesenteric thrombosis is a rare (0.3%), but life-threatening condition that can occur after bariatric and metabolic surgery due to increased hypercoagulability (Virchow's triad). Patients may present with non-specific abdominal pain, nausea, and vomiting. Given the nonspecific findings, diagnosis may be delayed. A contrasted CT scan provides the diagnosis and rules out other conditions. Management includes anticoagulation and potentially laparoscopic exploration depending on necrosis. [Question 120]

Reference: Goitein D, Matter I, Raziel A, et al. Portomesenteric Thrombosis Following Laparoscopic Bariatric Surgery: Incidence, Patterns of Clinical Presentation, and Etiology in a Bariatric Patient Population. JAMA Surg. 2013;148(4):340–346. doi:10.1001/jamasurg.2013.1053

285. (Content: I-B-8) In studying neurohormonal interactions, it is found that a specific second-order neuron within the paraventricular nucleus leads to decreased weight. This describes which of the following?

A. Proopiomelanocortin
B. Agouti-related peptide
C. Melanin-concentrating hormone
D. Alpha melanocyte-stimulating hormone

(D) The anorexigenic pathway comprises first-order neurons within the arcuate nucleus (POMC/CART neuron) and second-order neurons within the paraventricular nucleus (alpha-melanocyte-stimulating hormone and melanocortin 3 and 4 receptors). [Question 8]

Reference: Varela L, Horvath TL. Leptin and insulin pathways in POMC and AgRP neurons that modulate energy balance and glucose homeostasis. EMBO Rep. 2012;13(12):1079-1086. doi:10.1038/embor.2012.174

286. (Content: I-B-8) A patient is discussing his difficulty breaking an eating pattern that he has had for the past 5 years. The patient is a realtor and takes himself out to a steakhouse every time he sells a house. He has become more successful than when he first started and now is finding himself going out to eat multiple times per week. Which area of the brain is responsible for this eating pattern?

A. Limbic system
B. Hippocampus
C. Homeostatic center
D. Amygdala

(A) This patient is experiencing hedonic eating in which he eats as a reward for selling a home. Every time he sells a home and earns a steak for dinner, dopamine is released from the limbic system. This same reward system in the limbic system can also lead to addiction. [Question 37]

Reference: Farr OM, Li CR, Mantzoros CS. Central nervous system regulation of eating: Insights from human brain imaging. Metabolism. 2016 May;65(5):699-713. doi: 10.1016/j.metabol.2016.02.002. Epub 2016 Feb 6. PMID: 27085777; PMCID: PMC4834455.

287. (Content: III-D-1) When was lorcaserin (Belviq®) taken off the market and why?

    A. 1990 due to serotonin syndrome
    B. 1997 due to heart valve problems
    C. 2020 due to increased cancer risks
    D. 2022 due to increased risk of pancreatitis

(C) Lorcaserin (Belviq®), a serotonin 5-HT2C receptor agonist, was removed from the market in February 2020 due to an increased incidence of malignancy during a clinical trial. In contrast, fenfluramine combined with phentermine, termed "fen-phen," was taken off the market in 1997 due to the increased risk of valvular heart defects caused by fenfluramine (serotonin 5-HT2B receptor agonist).

Note: It is advised to know the year and reason that lorcaserin and phentermine-fenfluramine were removed from the market. [Question 156]

Reference: Up to Date: "Lorcaserin (United States: Withdrawn from market): Drug information"
Reference: Up to Date: "Valvular heart disease induced by drugs"

288. (Content: III-H-2) An 8-year-old female is diagnosed with Bardet-Biedl syndrome and a discussion of treatment options ensues. If started on setmelanotide, which of the following is a potential side effect?

    A. Nephrolithiasis
    B. Tachycardia
    C. Gastroparesis
    D. Skin hyperpigmentation

(D) Significant adverse reactions associated with setmelanotide include new or worsening depression or suicidal ideation, increased sexual arousal (labial hypersensitivity and priapism), and skin hyperpigmentation. In addition to its effects on the MC4R pathways associated with anorexic effects, setmelanotide may also stimulate MC1R skin receptors, which regulate skin pigmentation. [Question 184]

Reference: Setmelanotide package inserts.

289. (Content: III-F-4) Which of the following is most important prior to metabolic and bariatric surgery?

    A. Delay surgery until a HbA1c of <8% is maintained
    B. Adherence to a 6-month dietary plan
    C. Screen all surgical patients with a TSH
    D. Avoid hormonal therapy 3 weeks prior to surgery

(D) Estrogen-containing birth control should be held for one month and hormone replacement therapy 3 weeks prior to bariatric and metabolic surgery to reduce the risk of venous thrombosis. A TSH for screening is not recommended devoid of symptoms. Insurance-mandated weight loss requirements or arbitrary time-based approaches (e.g., 6 months of dieting) pre-operatively is not beneficial. Avoid post-operative hyperglycemia, however a specific hemoglobin A1c target pre-operatively should not delay surgery. [Question 182]

Reference: "ASMBS position statement on preoperative patient optimization before metabolic and bariatric surgery" Jonathan Carter, M.D., Julietta Chang, M.D., T. Javier Birriel, M.D., Fady Moustarah, M.D., et Al. Received 4 May 2021; accepted 27 August 2021

290. (Content: III-D-2) A 14-year-old female is on the maximum dose of phentermine/topiramate ER for weight loss and has lost 5% of her total body weight. Unfortunately, her father recently lost his job, including insurance coverage, and this medication is no longer affordable. Which of the following is a potential complication the daughter may experience if abruptly discontinued?

    A. Depression
    B. Seizure
    C. Rapid heartbeat
    D. Paresthesia

(B) With sudden discontinuation of topiramate, especially higher dosages, patients are at an increased risk of seizures. This medication should be tapered off, rather than stopped abruptly, to prevent this potential complication. [Question 105]

Reference: Phentermine/topiramate ER package insert

291. (Content: I-A-4) A 67-year-old male is following up from a motor vehicle accident in which the patient was ejected from the car, requiring emergent neurosurgery for a frontal epidural hematoma six months prior. The patient complains of erectile dysfunction, weight gain, frequent headaches, and cold intolerance since the accident. Which is the most likely cause of this patient's excess weight?

    A. Post-traumatic stress disorder
    B. Hypothalamic obesity
    C. Central hypothyroidism
    D. Hypogonadotropic hypogonadism

(B) Hypothalamic obesity occurs due to damage of the ventromedial hypothalamus (VMH), leading to loss of homeostatic inputs and thus causing decreased energy expenditure, hyperphagia, and subsequent obesity. Hypothalamic obesity can be caused by a craniopharyngioma, brain radiation, trauma, intracranial surgeries, increased intracranial pressure, or other brain tumors. These causes can occur in children as well. [Question 42]

Reference: Up To Date: "Obesity in adults: Etiologies and risk factors"

292. (Content: II-D-2) A patient is undergoing a bioelectrical impedance analysis at her initial obesity medicine consultation. Which of the following in her history would reduce the accuracy of this test?

    A. Eating food before the test
    B. Taking hydrochlorothiazide daily
    C. History of alcohol use disorder
    D. Exercising the day prior

(A) Bioelectrical impedance analysis is used to determine body fat composition. Limitations include accuracy at extremes of body mass index and inability to be performed if a cardiac device is implanted (MR spectroscopy should also be avoided if a cardiac pacemaker or defibrillator is present). Patients should be euvolemic and avoid exercising, alcohol, and food several hours before measurement for the most accurate results. [Question 50]

Reference: Kyle UG, Bosaeus I, De Lorenzo AD, Deurenberg P, Elia M, Gómez JM, Heitmann BL, Kent-Smith L, Melchior JC, Pirlich M, Scharfetter H, Schols AM, Pichard C; Composition of the ESPEN Working Group. Bioelectrical impedance analysis--part I: review of principles and methods. Clin Nutr. 2004 Oct;23(5):1226-43. doi: 10.1016/j.clnu.2004.06.004. PMID: 15380917.

293. (Content: III-F-5b) A 32-year-old female with a history of diabetes type II and obesity class I presents to the emergency department after experiencing a seizure. Her glucose level on arrival was 18 mg/dL (reference range: 70–110 mg/dL), which responded well to dextrose. She is post-ictal and cannot provide a medical history, however, her husband states she was recently prescribed tirzepatide. Which other medication was she most likely taking?

A. **Glipizide**
B. Sitagliptan
C. Semaglutide
D. Empagliflozin

(A) Although many of the weight-negative medications used to treat diabetes do not cause hypoglycemia themselves, when combined with hypoglycemic agents along with weight loss, hypoglycemia can occur. Sulfonylureas (e.g., glipizide) and insulin are the two most common medications that cause hypoglycemia. [Question 129]

Reference: Kim TY, Kim S, Schafer AL. Medical Management of the Postoperative Bariatric Surgery Patient. [Updated 2020 Aug 24]. In: Feingold KR, Anawalt B, Boyce A, et al., editors. Endotext [Internet]. South Dartmouth (MA): MDText.com, Inc.; 2000-. Available from: https://www.ncbi.nlm.nih.gov/books/NBK481901/

294. (Content: III-H-1) An 11-year-old female presents to the office for a well-child check. Her BMI is in the 90th percentile. She has no risk factors and otherwise feels well. What is the weight loss goal of this patient?

A. 1 lb weight loss per week
B. 2 lb weight loss per week
C. 1 lb weight loss per month
D. **Weight maintenance**

(D) Children with a BMI in the 85th-94th percentile with no evidence of health risks can safely be managed with prevention. If there are health risks, then start the 4-tiered system. Prevention and prevention plus (1st tier) promote weight maintenance because their BMI will decrease with increasing vertical height. [Question 169]

Reference: Expert Committee Recommendations Regarding the Prevention, Assessment, and Treatment of Child and Adolescent Overweight and Obesity: Summary Report and APPENDIX. Sarah E. Barlow and the Expert Committee; Pediatrics December 2007, 120 (Supplement 4) S164-S192; DOI: https://doi.org/10.1542/peds.2007-2329C.

295. (Content: I-B-5) A 24-year-old female presents to the clinic. She states she goes to bed at midnight and sleeps until 9 am. She is a computer programmer and sits at her computer for 8 hours, only taking a short break for lunch. She drinks 3 cups of coffee daily. Her only medical condition is hypothyroidism, treated with levothyroxine. Which of the following places her at an increased risk of cardiovascular disease?

A. **Career**
B. Sleep pattern
C. Hypothyroid disease
D. Coffee consumption

(A) Although this patient's career, in general, does not increase her risk of cardiovascular disease, her sedentary position associated with her career does. More than 3 hours of sedentary time increases the risk of cardiovascular disease. To minimize this risk, standing desks and more frequent breaks with physical movement can be beneficial. [Question 24]

Reference: Borodulin K, Kärki A, Laatikainen T, Peltonen M, Luoto R. Daily Sedentary Time and Risk of Cardiovascular Disease: The National FINRISK 2002 Study. J Phys Act Health. 2015 Jul;12(7):904-8. doi: 10.1123/jpah.2013-0364. Epub 2014 Aug 22. PMID: 25153761.

296. (Content: III-F-3) A 19-year-old male has undergone a Roux-en-Y gastric bypass seven months ago and returns for follow-up after having abdominal pain, nausea, and right shoulder pain after meals. He occasionally eats fast food for convenience but has reduced portions. He has lost 65 lbs (29.5 kg) since surgery. Which of the following is most likely the cause of his symptoms?

A. Anatomic ulceration
B. **Biliary colic**
C. Internal hernia
D. Small intestine bowel overgrowth

(B) Cholelithiasis can occur with any rapid weight loss. It can become symptomatic with nausea, vomiting, and right upper quadrant pain that may radiate to the shoulder. Eight percent of patients who have undergone gastric bypass require a cholecystectomy after surgery. [Question 119]

Reference: Up to Date: "Laparoscopic Roux-en-Y gastric bypass"

297. (Content: III-A-1) A 9-year-old male presents for a well-child check. His BMI is in the 92nd percentile. What would be the best way to discuss this with the patient?

A. Can you tell me what types of foods you like to eat?
B. **Would you mind if I ask you some questions about your body weight?**
C. I am concerned about your BMI. Is this something you have thought about?
D. How do you feel about discussing a dietary and exercise plan today?

(B) Before discussing a patient's weight, it is important to ask for permission. This is part of the 5 A's of obesity management (ask, assess, advise, agree, arrange/assist). [Question 147]

Reference: Obesity medicine association: Obesity Algorithm (2021)

298. (Content: II-D-3b) A 19-year-old female presents for a follow-up regarding polycystic ovarian syndrome (PCOS). A medical student asks the provider about the reason for decreased sex hormone binding globulin (SHBG) in this condition. What is the most accurate response?

A. **Hyperinsulinism decreases hepatic SHBG production**
B. Free androgens negatively feedback on estrogen production
C. Theca cells produce estrogen, which lowers SHBG levels
D. PCOS has high levels of SHBG, not low levels

(A) The rise in insulin resistance is not fully understood in PCOS, however this resistance causes beta cells in the pancreas to increase insulin production. Hyperinsulinism inhibits the hepatic production of SHBG and increases the production of androgens via theca cell stimulation, leading to elevated levels of free androgens and is the reason for virilization. [Question 91]

Reference: Zhu JL, Chen Z, Feng WJ, Long SL, Mo ZC. Sex hormone-binding globulin and polycystic ovary syndrome. Clin Chim Acta. 2019 Dec;499:142-148. doi: 10.1016/j.cca.2019.09.010. Epub 2019 Sep 13. PMID: 31525346.
Reference: Up To Date: "Epidemiology, phenotype, and genetics of the polycystic ovary syndrome in adults"

299. (Content: III-D-1) Of the following medications used for weight loss, which is most likely to have an adverse effect on blood pressure?

A. Naltrexone
B. Phentermine
C. Bupropion
D. Topiramate

(C) Bupropion has been shown to have an adverse effect on blood pressure despite its improvements with weight loss. Importantly, phentermine has not demonstrated a significant increase in heart rate or systolic/diastolic blood pressure in most patients, although some patients may be more susceptible. [Question 162]

Reference: Hendricks EJ, Greenway FL, Westman EC, Gupta AK. Blood pressure and heart rate effects, weight loss and maintenance during long-term phentermine pharmacotherapy for obesity. Obesity (Silver Spring). 2011 Dec;19(12):2351-60. doi: 10.1038/oby.2011.94. Epub 2011 Apr 28. PMID: 21527891.
Reference: Bupropion package insert

300. (Content: III-A-2) A 21-year-old female is trying to quit smoking before she becomes pregnant. She has unreliable transportation and the nearest location to purchase cigarettes is two miles away. During your discussions, it is recommended to no longer purchase cartons of cigarettes but rather buy only one pack at a time. What behavioral therapy component is this?

A. Goal setting
B. Stimulus control
C. Reward
D. Self-monitoring

(B) In this situation, the patient's barrier to cigarettes is transportation. Using the unreliable transportation to her advantage, thereby limiting the convenience by not purchasing a carton at a time, makes it much more challenging to get cigarettes. This is the idea behind stimulus control, making it more difficult or "out of reach" to get instant gratification. Similar to alcohol or tobacco cessation techniques, cognitive behavioral therapy can be utilized for weight loss. Avoiding the purchasing of unhealthy foods and bringing them into the home inhibits the availability of the stimuli. [Question 127]

Reference: Dalle Grave R, Centis E, Marzocchi R, El Ghoch M, Marchesini G. Major factors for facilitating change in behavioral strategies to reduce obesity. Psychol Res Behav Manag. 2013;6:101-110. Published 2013 Oct 3. doi:10.2147/PRBM.S40460

Test Content Outline and
Answer List Summary

I. Basic Concepts – 25%

A. Determinants of Obesity
    1. Lifestyle/Behavioral
    2. Environmental/Cultural
    3. Genetic
    4. Secondary
    5. Epigenetics and Fetal Environment

B. Physiology/Pathophysiology
    1. Neurohormonal
    2. Enterohormonal/Microbiota
    3. Body Fat Distribution
    4. Pathophysiology of Obesity-Related Disorders/Comorbidities
    5. Body Composition and Energy Expenditure
    6. Energy Balance and Hormonal Adaptation to Weight Loss
    7. Obesity Related Cell Physiology and Metabolism
    8. Brain, Gut, Adipocyte Interaction

C. Epidemiology
    1. Incidence and Prevalence, Demographic Distribution
    2. Across the Life Cycle

D. General Concepts of Nutrition
    1. Macro and Micronutrients
    2. Gastrointestinal Sites of Nutrient Absorption
    3. Obesity Related Vitamin and Mineral Metabolism
    4. Macronutrient Diet Composition and Effects on Body Weight and Metabolism

E. General Concepts of Physical Activity
    1. Biomechanics and kinesiology
    2. Cardiorespiratory Fitness and Body Composition

II. Diagnosis and Evaluation – 30%

A. History
- 1. Medications
- 2. Family History
- 3. Comorbidities/Assessment and evaluation
- 4. Sleep

B. Lifestyle/Behavior/Psychosocial
- 1. Demographic/Socioeconomic/Cultural/ Lifestyle/Occupational
- 2. Physical Activity
- 3. Nutrition/Diet
- 4. Eating Disorders/Disordered Eating
- 5. Body image disturbance

C. Physical Assessment
- 1. BMI
- 2. Waist Circumference
- 3. Physical Findings of obesity and Comorbid Conditions
- 4. Vital Signs
- 5. Underlying Syndromes
- 6. Signs of Nutritional Deficiency
- 7. Growth indices

D. Procedures and Laboratory Testing
- 1. Resting Metabolic Rate
- 2. Body Composition Analysis
- 3. Diagnostic Tests
    - a. Comorbidities
    - b. Secondary Obesity

E. Screening Questionnaires
F. Research Tools

III. Treatment – 40%

A. Behavior
    1. Behavioral Counseling Techniques/Therapies
    2. Self-Monitoring Techniques/Tools
B. Diet
    1. Calorie and Micro/Macronutrient
    2. Very Low Calorie Diet
    3. Meal Replacements
    4. Effect on Comorbid Conditions
C. Physical Activity
    1. Prescription
    2. Mechanisms of Action
    3. Effect on Comorbid Conditions
D. Pharmacotherapy, Pharmacology and Pharmacokinetics
    1. Risks, Benefits, and Adverse Effects
    2. Indications/Contraindications
    3. Monitoring and Follow Up
    4. Prescription Dose and Frequency
    5. Drug-Drug, Drug-Nutrient, Drug-Herbal Interactions
    6. Off Label Usage/Over-the-counter (OTC)
    7. Multi-drug/Combination Therapy
    8. Management of Drug-Induced Weight Gain
    9. Effect on Comorbid Conditions
E. Alternative, Emerging, and Investigational Therapies
F. Surgical Procedures
    1. Types, Risks, Benefits
    2. Indications and Contraindications
    3. Complications
    4. Pre-operative Assessment and Preparation
    5. Post-operative Management
        a. Medical Inpatient
        b. Medical Outpatient
        c. Nutritional
    6. Adolescent Surgery
    7. Effect on Comorbid Conditions

G. Strategies
      1. Age-Related Treatment
      2. Risks Associated with Excessive Weight Loss
      3. Management of Weight Plateau
      4. Prevention of Obesity and Weight Gain
      5. Management of Comorbid Conditions During Weight Loss
      6. Effect of Weight Loss on Comorbid Conditions
      7. Treatment of Comorbid Conditions

H. Pediatric obesity
      1. Treatment Guidelines
      2. Pharmacotherapy
      3. Bariatric Surgery
      4. Family Support and Participation

IV. Practice Management – 5%

A. Patient care Issues
    1. Weight Bias, Stigma/Discrimination
    2. Culturally Tailored Communication
    3. Ethics
B. Office Procedures
    1. Policies and Protocols
    2. Adult Obesity Management Guidelines and Recommendations
    3. Physician Personal Health Behaviors
    4. Online and remote management tools
C. Interdisciplinary Team
D. Advocacy/Public Health
E. Other
    1. Cost Effectiveness of Treatment Options
    2. Awareness of Societal Cost of Obesity
    3. Reimbursement and Coding

Content breakdown per life cycle:

- Pediatric and adolescent content: 15%
- Adult content: 20%
- Content relevant to all life cycles: 65%

Answers

	Practice Test 1		Practice Test 2		Practice Test 3	
1. A	26. A	51. C	76. C	101. B	126. D
2. A	27. C	52. B	77. C	102. B	127. B
3. B	28. A	53. D	78. C	103. D	128. C
4. A	29. B	54. A	79. C	104. C	129. D
5. D	30. A	55. D	80. B	105. A	130. D
6. B	31. C	56. B	81. B	106. A	131. A
7. B	32. D	57. C	82. D	107. C	132. A
8. D	33. B	58. A	83. B	108. A	133. D
9. D	34. B	59. A	84. C	109. B	134. D
10. C	35. D	60. C	85. A	110. C	135. C
11. A	36. A	61. A	86. D	111. B	136. C
12. A	37. A	62. D	87. A	112. D	137. C
13. C	38. C	63. B	88. C	113. B	138. A
14. A	39. A	64. C	89. A	114. B	139. C
15. C	40. B	65. B	90. A	115. A	140. A
16. C	41. D	66. A	91. D	116. B	141. B
17. A	42. A	67. D	92. D	117. C	142. D
18. D	43. C	68. A	93. B	118. A	143. A
19. A	44. D	69. C	94. C	119. C	144. C
20. A	45. A	70. C	95. B	120. A	145. D
21. C	46. B	71. D	96. C	121. C	146. A
22. B	47. D	72. C	97. D	122. C	147. B
23. C	48. A	73. A	98. C	123. D	148. C
24. C	49. D	74. C	99. D	124. B	149. B
25. A	50. C	75. B	100. D	125. D	150. B

Answers

Practice Test 4		Practice Test 5		Practice Test 6	
151. B	176. B	201. A	226. B	251. A	276. A
152. C	177. D	202. A	227. C	252. A	277. B
153. A	178. C	203. B	228. A	253. D	278. A
154. D	179. A	204. C	229. A	254. A	279. D
155. B	180. C	205. C	230. C	255. A	280. D
156. D	181. B	206. D	231. C	256. A	281. B
157. C	182. B	207. D	232. B	257. C	282. C
158. B	183. C	208. B	233. C	258. C	283. B
159. A	184. C	209. B	234. B	259. B	284. B
160. C	185. C	210. A	235. B	260. A	285. D
161. D	186. A	211. D	236. C	261. B	286. A
162. A	187. A	212. B	237. B	262. C	287. C
163. D	188. B	213. B	238. D	263. B	288. D
164. A	189. B	214. A	239. C	264. C	289. D
165. D	190. C	215. B	240. B	265. D	290. B
166. D	191. C	216. B	241. B	266. B	291. B
167. C	192. A	217. D	242. B	267. A	292. A
168. C	193. C	218. A	243. C	268. A	293. A
169. D	194. D	219. B	244. C	269. B	294. D
170. C	195. D	220. B	245. D	270. B	295. A
171. D	196. B	221. D	246. C	271. B	296. B
172. C	197. B	222. B	247. D	272. B	297. B
173. B	198. A	223. A	248. A	273. C	298. A
174. C	199. D	224. A	249. A	274. B	299. C
175. A	200. B	225. C	250. C	275. B	300. B

Provide Feedback After the Exam

Be entered to win a $100 Amazon gift card!

Drawing October 29th, 2023. Five winners will be chosen.
Constructive and detailed feedback appreciated.